"What I appreciate most about *Helping Your Child with Extreme Picky Eating* is its respectful approach for both parents and children. It offers parents hope, understanding, and practical strategies that really work. Based on sound research and a true understanding of children, it gently but confidently guides families through the steps of building a healthy relationship with food."

—**Mary Sheedy Kurcinka, EdD**, licensed teacher, parent educator, and author of *Raising Your Spirited Child*

"Finally, an antidote to the infuriating trend of books about tricking children into eating. Rowell and McGlothlin expertly illuminate the complex emotional world of children with extreme picky eating and the caregivers who struggle to feed them. *Helping Your Child with Extreme Picky Eating* is a masterpiece of practical strategies, compassion, and reassurance that's perfect for parents, pediatricians, and anyone who remembers hating 'just one more bite.'"

—**Jessica Setnick, MS, RD, CEDRD**, pediatric eating disorder specialist, cofounder of the International Federation of Eating Disorder Dietitians, and author of *The Eating Disorders Clinical Pocket Guide*

"With the persistent challenge of classification and treatment of feeding problems, eating disorder professionals are increasingly charged with treating children with feeding difficulties, avoidant/restrictive food intake disorder (ARFID) cases, and selective eating. This book is an invaluable resource for eating disorder (ED) professionals in need of a thorough introduction to the spectrum of selective eating issues that may be outside their primary area of expertise, from typical 'picky' eating to more pervasive food aversions. The authors' expert handling of this topic will empower both professionals and parents to better understand and support their selective eaters."

—**Katherine Zavodni, MPH, RD, LDN,** registered
dietitian specializing in outpatient nutrition therapy for
eating disorders, family nutrition and childhood feeding,
and intuitive eating

"*Helping Your Child with Extreme Picky Eating* is a practical, child-focused, and guilt-free guide to addressing a variety of eating challenges. This book respects and values the parent as an expert. The nonjudgmental approach and easy-to-follow techniques will empower parents to make family mealtime a positive experience. By providing a sound overview of feeding development, Rowell and McGlothlin changed my understanding of typical eating. The suggested scripts and keen insight into the child's perspective takes the guesswork out of applying the STEPS+. I walked away with a deeper understanding of how children experience feeding and how my own 'feeding temperament' affects how I relate to my children around food. Short-order cooking is out the door and dessert is on the table with dinner now. We're all enjoying a happier mealtime! My only wish is that I'd had this book when my children were babies. I would strongly recommend this book to any parent who is struggling with mealtime."

—**Erin Erickson, MPH, MN, RN,** founder and cohost
of Mom Enough®

"Katja Rowell and Jenny McGlothlin *get* the anxiety and many challenges both children and families feel when children are highly selective eaters! They offer sensitive, thoughtful, and practical suggestions to support families in their journey toward happier and healthier mealtimes."

—**Marsha Dunn Klein, MEd, OTR/L, FAOTA**, pediatric therapist, educator, author, and co-owner of Mealtime Connections, a pediatric therapy clinic in Tucson, AZ

"Lots of books promise to help solve 'picky eating' problems, but this one actually does! Rowell and McGlothlin have put together a comprehensive masterpiece."

—**Skye Van Zetten**, blogger at mealtimehostage.com

"Finally! Not just an acknowledgment, but an exploration and even a 'how-to manual' on dealing with the long-neglected missing piece of pediatric feeding therapy—the emotional dynamic for both the child and the parent! Let's face it, eating is not just about nutrition. It's also about enjoyment and family relationships. This gets lost amidst health and medical concerns when a child severely limits his eating. Katja Rowell and Jenny McGlothlin have given us a map for restoring and healing these components as well. Parents and therapists alike will be profoundly grateful."

—**Jennifer Meyer, MA, CCC-SLP,** cocreator of care-to-collaborate.com, and popular international speaker in the areas of pediatric dysphagia and neonatal therapy

"Finally, there's a solid resource for families who struggle with extreme picky eating! Rowell and McGlothlin leave no stone unturned as they help parents navigate all aspects of their child's eating, from the 'how' of family dinners to decisions about feeding therapy. I will recommend this book again and again."

> —**Maryann Jacobsen, MS, RD**, author, blogger, speaker,
> and coauthor of *Fearless Feeding*

"A wonderful, parent-friendly resource that is easy to read and full of practical suggestions to help your child 'come to the table!'"

> —**Catherine S. Shaker, MS/CCC-SLP, BCS-S**, pediatric
> speech-language pathologist at the Florida Hospital for
> Children in Orlando, FL, and coauthor of "The Early
> Feeding Skills Assessment Tool for NICU Infants"

"*Helping Your Child with Extreme Picky Eating* is wonderful! I currently work with a young male client who struggles with eating, and I can honestly say that this information is so crucial for even mental health therapists who are working to help families dealing with feeding issues. I wish all school counselors could have access to this material. The material in this book has assisted me in helping my client's family in a way that I was struggling to before reading! Thank you for writing this tremendously helpful text!"

> —**Christine J. Schimmel, EdD, NCC, LPC**, assistant
> professor of counseling at West Virginia University and
> author of numerous texts and articles on impact therapy,
> a multisensory, creative approach to counseling and
> group counseling

Helping Your Child *with* Extreme Picky Eating

A Step-by-Step Guide
for Overcoming Selective
Eating, Food Aversion,
and Feeding Disorders

KATJA ROWELL, MD
JENNY M^CGLOTHLIN, MS, SLP

New Harbinger Publications, Inc.

Publisher's Note

This publication is designed to provide accurate and authoritative information in regard to the subject matter covered. It is sold with the understanding that the publisher is not engaged in rendering psychological, financial, legal, or other professional services. If expert assistance or counseling is needed, the services of a competent professional should be sought.

Medical Disclaimer

This book and the information it contains are provided for educational purposes only. The text of this book is not meant or intended to replace careful observation, evaluation, diagnosis, or ongoing medical or nutritional care for a child, and the text of this book should not be used in place of such careful observation, evaluation, diagnosis, or ongoing care. The authors have provided general information in this book and cannot make any assurances in regard to the applicability of any information to any particular person in any particular set of circumstances. The reader assumes all risk of taking any action or making any decision based on the information contained in this book. The authors shall have no liability or responsibility for any such action taken or decision made by any reader of this book, and no liability for any loss, injury, damage, or impairment allegedly arising from the information provided in this book.

Distributed in Canada by Raincoast Books

Copyright © 2015 by Katja Rowell and Jenny McGlothlin
New Harbinger Publications, Inc.
5674 Shattuck Avenue
Oakland, CA 94609
www.newharbinger.com

Cover design by Amy Shoup; Acquired by Jess O'Brien; Edited by Clancy Drake

Library of Congress Cataloging-in-Publication Data on file

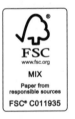
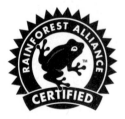

FSC
www.fsc.org
MIX
Paper from responsible sources
FSC® C011935

Printed in the United States of America

21   20   19

15   14   13   12   11   10   9   8

To the parents: May this book bring you hope, reassurance, and concrete strategies to help your child and family.

Thank you: To my daughter, a funny and entertaining dinner companion and general joy to be around. To my husband, best friend, love, camping partner, and dishwasher, for your unfailing support. To my parents, for wonderful meals and memories around the table growing up. And to my coauthor Jenny, a brilliant colleague, diagnostician, and friend.

Katja Rowell

I dedicate this labor of love to my three children, Kaden, Whitt, and Sydney, who keep me on my toes and make life a lovely adventure; my husband, Kyle, my loyal and level-headed partner in life, meals, and the logistics of three kids; my parents, who taught me the joy of food and family; and Katja, who inspires me on a daily basis with her devotion, compassion, and insight.

Jenny McGlothlin

Contents

Acknowledgments

We are grateful to those who taught and supported us along the way: Suzanne Evans Morris, for pioneering therapy within a trusting feeding relationship, and for believing in this book and writing the foreword for it; Ellyn Satter, whose groundbreaking work and division of responsibility are the foundation for relational and responsive feeding; and Hydee Becker, for her nutrition expertise and feeding wisdom.

Thank you to the following for their support and feedback on drafts of this book: Stephanie Larson, Skye Van Zetten, Michelle Gorman, Michelle Allison, David Bell, Rachel Wehner, Elizabeth Jackson, Pam Estes, Patty Morse, Katharine Zavodni, and Carol Danaher. Thanks to the University of Texas at Dallas Callier Center for Communication Disorders for their support and belief in the STEPS program. Thanks to Bora Chung, Jill Jones, and Kim Fiser for research and bibliography assistance, and to the designers of the Growth app (http://www.growthapp.net, used to generate the charts in this book) for a useful tool for tracking growth.

Foreword

by Suzanne Evans Morris, PhD

Most parents assume that feeding is a simple and natural aspect of nurturing and raising their children. When their child refuses food, doesn't want to eat, or eats an extremely limited variety of foods, they are both shocked and afraid. If you are a parent of an extremely picky eater, you may find yourself frightened that your child will not grow and develop normally. If you are a therapist working with families on feeding issues, you have probably seen parents respond emotionally to their belief that there is something wrong with them as parents when their child has problems with eating.

Responding to feeding issues with fear and a desire to control is understandable. From our earliest childhood experiences of "feeding" baby dolls and "fixing" toy cars, we learn that "a good mommy can feed her baby" and that "a good daddy can fix anything." Parents of a child with extreme picky eating have been primed to try everything they can think of to "get their child to eat." When their efforts to help their child don't fix the problem, they feel they've failed as parents— not understanding that feeding strategies that come from fear and from efforts to control are doomed to fail.

Helping Your Child with Extreme Picky Eating provides valuable guidance for parents whose children have feeding challenges, as well as for therapists working with those parents and children. And besides being an invaluable resource for parents of children whose picky eating issues create a deep concern for families, the book provides a template and tools for helping any child who experiences feeding and mealtime difficulties. The authors' aim is to support parents in building their children's positive relationship with food and mealtimes, so that the child becomes able to respond to her own internal cues around food. This kind of "inner directedness" is at the heart of healthy eating.

Many books and therapy programs address the reasons why a child becomes a picky eater. And learning how the stage is set for a child's need to say no to food—whether through difficulties in the feeding relationship, sensory processing and motor coordination issues, oral skill development, or medical challenges—can be extremely helpful for parents. However, most such books and programs lack real guidance on how to build eating desire and competence from the inside out, whatever a child's current eating situation. Rather, they depend on techniques to improve feeding skills or to manage the child's eating behavior. They do not address respectful ways that build upon every child's innate ability to be nourished physically and emotionally while enjoying mealtimes and food.

The STEPS+ approach presented in *Helping Your Child with Extreme Picky Eating* acknowledges that a child's feeding choices are often guided by unique physical, sensory, and emotional needs and fears, which can be addressed through established therapeutic feeding approaches. Traditional feeding therapy, however, is often centered on the knowledge and needs of parents and therapists. It fails to support the essential mealtime partnership and relationship between parent and child. Children whose needs and fears are understood, respected, and addressed begin to perceive the world differently and initiate changes when eating is built upon the foundation of a mealtime partnership that respects and honors both child and parent. The insight that trust, relationship, and partnership are central to feeding a child draws from the work of Ellyn Satter, a dietitian and family therapist who developed and has written extensively about the *division of responsibility in feeding,* or DOR. Satter's approach states that parents are responsible for the *what, where,* and *when* of meals, and children are responsible for *whether* and *how much* they eat of the food that is served. Mounting research supports the principle that when children are given a clear structure and trusted to make personal decisions about eating, they will begin to get in touch with their natural appetite and develop the confidence they need to eat based on hunger and a desire to participate in mealtimes, rather than engage in avoidance and power struggles.

As effective as the division of responsibility has been with typically developing children and their families, therapists have been slow to incorporate its principles when working with children with significant eating issues—what the authors of this book call "extreme picky eating." When children's feeding issues include a medical or neurological diagnosis, treatment typically focuses on medical, behavioral, or sensorimotor approaches. Certainly the parents of such children may feel they can only dream of letting their child eat—or not eat—as she chooses. The prospect is just too terrifying. Combining insights and approaches that fit each child and family, however, can lead to successful and happy mealtimes for everyone.

Helping Your Child with Extreme Picky Eating offers a perfect union of relational insights and understanding with deep therapeutic knowledge and many practical strategies that empower parents to help their children where it's needed most—in the home—and in the presence of even serious eating challenges. Katja Rowell and Jenny McGlothlin have crafted a book that provides very specific suggestions to help parents both understand and address their picky child's eating challenges. It belongs in the library of every parent or therapist who wants to support a child's (and a family's) positive relationship with food and mealtimes.

Introduction

Parenting a child with extreme picky eating can feel like running an endless marathon. Nothing about food and your child feels right: you fret about what to put on the table; you worry about nutrition and growth; your child can't go to camp because of his limited menu. He worries, panics, or has tantrums around new foods or eating in new places, or dinner is forty-five minutes of "hostage negotiation," as one mom put it. Whatever the circumstances, if your child's eating is affecting his social, emotional, or physical development and causing family conflict or worry, this book is for you.

You've probably encountered plenty of unhelpful advice. It doesn't help when your child's teacher insists *she* will get your child to eat oranges, or when the doctor's orders to "starve him out" haven't worked. Facebook photos of your niece devouring kale chips make you feel worse, and Internet support groups are full of conflicting, misleading, and disapproving comments—often everything but support. Lucky mothers of omnivores opine that Goldfish crackers— one of the few foods your child readily eats—are "toxic." You may have "failed" at creating a little foodie, "failed" at feeding therapy, or even been told your child has "failure to thrive," which is like a knife to the heart—because when you have a child, your job from day one is to nurture and feed. So what happens when feeding is such a struggle that it feels like your only options are to fight over every bite, or to surrender and serve his few accepted foods day after day, year after year?

This book is not about finding the one trick or rule that will "work." Rather, it's about a shift in how you approach feeding. It's about turning "failure" around and supporting your whole family while helping your child be able to enjoy a variety of foods in the right amounts so he can grow in a healthy way. It's about ending the battles over food, and looking forward to family dinners—maybe for the first time! It's about celebrating and enjoying your child, no matter what his challenges are, and not letting his eating define his life or your family's. Our wish is for all children to grow up healthy and happy, eating to the best of their abilities, and feeling good about food and their bodies.

Parenting a "Picky" Eater

Your child may have been labeled a "selective eater," a "problem feeder," "neophobic" (afraid of the new), "food aversive," or "failure to thrive." Maybe he's been diagnosed with a feeding disorder, or no longer needs a feeding tube but still struggles. He may eat only thirty foods, or only ten; or maybe there are only three *safe foods* that he is likely to eat and manages easily. (The preschooler who refuses anything but pureed peas, pears, and pretzels has three safe foods.)

What the Labels Mean

Problem feeder: A child who eats fewer than twenty foods, drops foods without adding others, eats different foods than the rest of the family, avoids entire food groups (like meats and vegetables), or becomes upset around new foods is often labeled a *problem feeder*.

Selective eating disorder: Similar definition to problem feeder. Not officially a diagnosis in adults or children; increasingly used to describe a limited range of accepted foods and refusal of unfamiliar foods.

Food aversion: May emerge after unpleasant experiences including illness, trauma, or choking; also generalized fear or anxiety around food. Often occurs with selective eating disorder or among problem feeders.

Neophobia: Fear of new things. Toddlers typically experience a phase of suspicion with new and even familiar foods, but extreme negative reactions to new foods may be labeled *neophobia*.

ARFID: Avoidant/restrictive food intake disorder, previously called *infantile anorexia*. The *Diagnostic and Statistical Manual of Mental Disorders* (DSM-5) defines it as starting before age six, lasting longer than one month, and characterized by an inability to take in enough nutrition orally for optimal growth, with a negative impact on weight and/or psychosocial functioning. There are three ARFID subgroups: sensory, little or no appetite, and aversive.

Failure to thrive: Inadequate physical growth. Often defined as weight below the fifth percentile; however, clinicians have used cutoffs at the tenth, fifth, or first percentile, or when growth slows significantly.

Feeding disorder: According to the American Speech-Language-Hearing Association, describes problems gathering food in the mouth and sucking, chewing, or swallowing for appropriate intake.

Currently there is no agreed-upon classification system that captures the complexity of pediatric feeding problems. In this book, we use the descriptor our clients use most, *extreme picky eating,* or EPE, which encompasses the various terms. (Note that we use the word "picky" to describe the child's eating, never to judge the child.) "Extreme picky eating" describes the limited variety of accepted foods or the limited amounts *and* considers the way the child behaves around and relates to food.

Among our readers may be parents whose child has never taken a bite of food, and parents whose child has twenty or more accepted foods. Some parents would be thrilled if their child ate ice cream for dinner; for others, that would disappoint. Keep in mind the range of experiences your fellow parents deal with, and adapt the advice in this book to your situation.

Whatever your child's situation, you are not alone. One in three parents identifies her child as "picky," and up to 80 percent of children with developmental delays struggle with eating. Various sources report that 3 to 25 percent of American children have feeding challenges. Based on our research, conversations with colleagues, and experience, we believe the prevalence is around 10 to 15 percent. Taking into account census data, that's four to six million American children under age ten with extreme picky eating! Even famous foodie Michael Pollan had a food neophobic son who "only ate white food" (Beers 2009).

Not only are you not alone; it's also not your fault. It's not your fault if your child is highly intelligent or wildly independent, has a cautious temperament or developmental delays, is on the autism spectrum, is especially sensitive to flavors, or avoids certain textures; these factors are beyond your control. Some parents believe their children struggle because they are *supertasters*—able to sense bitter tastes and other flavors more intensely—and studies suggest that about a quarter of the population are supertasters (Bartoshuk, Duffy, and Miller 1994). While supertasting can play a role, many selective eaters are not supertasters, and many supertasters enjoy a wide variety of foods. According to Bartoshuk and colleagues (1994), about a quarter of the population may be *nontasters*, with fewer taste buds and less ability to taste. We theorize that a lack of pleasure from dulled flavors may also play an as-yet unexplored role in picky eating. Complex stuff!

Many factors contribute to the problem of extreme picky eating in ways we don't yet understand, but a critical piece of the puzzle is the interaction between parent and child around food. It is not the therapist or some combination of texture and flavor that will make the most difference. *You* are the critical factor in developing a healthier feeding relationship with your child. This is a tender point, as parents tend to blame themselves for difficulties in the feeding relationship, so we'll say it again—it's not your fault. Rather, when a child has eating challenges, poor support and advice set parents up for feeding interactions that make initial problems worse. The reverse is also true: good guidance and support help you and your child move past feeding difficulties together.

Too many families lose hope and resign themselves to serving a handful of accepted foods. When things get really stressful, parents don't care how many vegetables or bites their child eats—*if he eats happily.* Reaching that goal means going beyond working on oral motor skills or getting your child to eat two bites. It's understandably frustrating when years after completing "successful" therapy (thought of as avoiding tube-feeding) parents still can't see the path to more normal eating.

With the tried and tested steps in this book, you'll gain a better understanding of your child's challenges and why past strategies failed. You'll be empowered to guide your child to greater comfort with, and enjoyment of, a wider variety of foods. We aim to clearly define that path, without sacrificing your child's emotional, social, or physical health.

Don't give up, and don't despair. We see kids make incredible improvements all the time. And it's also worth noting that adult selective eaters can be healthy and lead fulfilling, happy lives. As one selective-eating dad explained, "I have a wonderful wife, amazing kids, and a job I like. I play basketball and my health is great; I just don't like vegetables. I want my kids to have a shot at liking more foods, but I'm pretty happy. That calms me down about my son's eating." You can help your child eat well, and the first step is to understand why you are struggling.

Building a Foundation of Understanding

This book is structured to give you a strong foundation of understanding to prepare you for the strategies (or steps) that follow, allowing you to learn to confidently handle daily decisions around food. Each chapter builds on the last, and we suggest you read from beginning to end before making significant changes. Chapter 1 reviews typical development around growth and eating, preparing you to explore, in chapter 2, challenges your child may bring to the table. Chapter 3 explains how you may have found yourself stuck in unpleasant and counterproductive feeding patterns.

Chapters 4 through 8 are organized around the five basic components of our STEPS+ (Supportive Treatment of Eating in PartnershipS) approach:

Step 1: Decrease stress, anxiety, and power struggles (chapter 4).

Step 2: Establish a routine (chapter 5).

Step 3: Enjoy pleasant family meals (chapter 6).

Step 4: Build skills in "what" and "how" to feed (chapter 7).

Step 5: Strengthen and support oral motor and sensory skills (chapter 8).

Chapter 9 helps you understand what progress looks like in both the short and long term; it will look different for every child and family. More resources and support are available on the website associated with this book, http://www.newharbinger.com/31106, including handouts for teachers and childcare providers, a log for tracking feeding and intake, information about apps for charting your child's growth, and more.

The focus of the STEPS+ approach is on reestablishing trust—and it won't feel like therapy. It helps you create structured routine and optimize your child's appetite so he learns (or relearns) to eat a healthy amount. Your confidence around menu planning, food modification, and making the family table an enjoyable place will improve. You will discover strategies and ideas to support your child's oral motor and sensory skills at home, as well as an overview of therapeutic options to help you decide whether to pursue therapy and, if so, how to find the right help. Finally, you will learn to identify progress, and we will share encouraging words from other parents.

As you read, you may notice some repetition of concepts. Decreasing your child's anxiety improves her appetite and lessens power struggles, and so does routine. We separate the steps for clarity, but together they maximize success.

Note that we refer more to "moms," because our experience is that primarily mothers accompany children to therapy, seek phone support, or read the books. We don't mean to diminish the importance of dads. Dads, your contribution is critical, and we love when both parents are involved. Also note that identifying details have been changed for the children and scenarios described, and we alternate between "he" and "she" when referring to children in the abstract.

Addressing Your Concerns and Dilemmas

Here is a sampling of some of the most common questions we'll address:

What do I do if she doesn't eat dinner but wants a snack as soon as I've cleared everything away? (chapter 5)

How do I wean him off the iPad that we've had at the table for years? (chapter 8)

I dread eating out with my child. Is it okay to bring some of his safe foods? (chapter 6)

Parents tell us that having ideas about what to say (or not say) when faced with an upset child is most helpful. Therefore, we include **suggested scripts** for common scenarios, **bolded** for reference. Use them word for word, or find what works for you. "Food for Thought" questions, another running feature in the book, help you understand and empathize with your child. Tips and exercises throughout the chapters reinforce skills and are an excellent way to include other caregivers.

Benefits for the Whole Family

Parents with children in therapy often complain that siblings' (and their own) needs fall away as therapy tasks distort or destroy family meals. What you will learn throughout this book (outside of specific skills in chapter 8) applies to all your children, whether or not they have eating challenges or are smaller or larger than average.

Your child with picky eating *and* her siblings will improve when you allow *all* your children to eat *according to their own body signals* (though how much and what they eat probably won't look the same from child to child). We've even had clients say, "My husband tries new things since I stopped pushing!" And in spite of their increasing independence, teens also benefit from routine and pressure-free, respectful family meals.

Skills for a Lifetime

Although this book is geared toward children aged roughly two to eight, the basic principles, philosophies, and skills apply across all ages. If you have a tween or older child, some questions and exercises may not directly apply. However, when appropriate, content is adapted to the older or younger child, and reflection on any of the questions or exercises can provide insight, as many readers will have struggled since their children were infants.

If You're Waiting for an Evaluation or Therapy Appointment

Waiting for an evaluation is agonizing if your child is struggling. In the meantime, STEPS+ supports your child's eating and helps you recognize what *not* to do. You may even see so much progress that you cancel that appointment! It's happened. If you continue with compatible therapies (see chapter 8), these strategies, and the philosophies behind them, will be key to progress at home and in therapy.

Choosing What to Serve

Because we believe that *how* children are fed is the key to what they eat, we wait to address *what* foods to serve until late in the book. Without establishing pleasant meals and routine and reducing your child's anxiety, you can cook a thousand things and never find the perfect recipe. Your child's attitude and anxiety must improve before you can expect her to explore new foods. But we understand you need to put food on the table every day. So while you work on the steps, we suggest you continue serving what you are serving now. Work on the "what" when you feel ready, which may be early in the process, or not until you have established regular family meals.

Discovering There Are Many Ways to Do It "Right"

A key feature of STEPS+ is that you don't have to implement every strategy right away. One mother found that jumping into routine meals and snacks, serving family-style, *and* turning off the iPad overwhelmed her son, and he ate almost nothing for three days. On her next try, she stuck with structure and family meals but allowed the iPad. This slower approach eased the transition for her son (who has mild autism), increasing his comfort with and interest in different foods. She was excited by the progress he'd made, but still felt guilty for "not doing it right." However, doing it right differs for every family, so say no to guilt or thinking you or your child should be progressing differently or more quickly.

Making changes around the way you feed your child might feel really different at first. It was a hard adjustment for one dad who, after years of rules and protocols, felt as if he had been feeding his child on an "alien planet," slowly working his way back to Earth. For others, change is a relief. One mother shared, "This feels so much better than fighting over every bite."

Learning to Trust Your Gut

Parents often lament that what they were told to do to get their child to eat felt wrong, but, "They're the experts, right?" Wrong! *You* are your child's expert. If your gut tells you that what you're trying isn't helping, and you dread mealtimes, then it most likely *is* the wrong approach. If requiring your child to take one bite of everything on his plate (often called the *one-bite rule*) causes epic battles, or therapy protocols lead to tears and gagging, it undermines your child's trust in you. This in turn undermines progress and his relationship with food.

Let the way you feel guide you in supporting your child's progress. Parents who don't feel good about food or their own bodies may feel as if they can't trust their gut when it comes to feeding. The steps will help. If you find yourself dreading meals less, noticing smiles appearing at the table, and beginning to feel a sense of *relief*...trust that. Let positive interactions build your faith in the process. If you've tried different strategies and therapies, you may feel jaded. You might not trust *us* yet, and that's okay. Keep an open mind along the way.

Our Path to STEPS+

I (Katja) didn't learn about feeding during my medical training or when I was a family doctor (giving feeding advice!). I learned about feeding as a parent when I realized I felt confident about *what* to feed but not *how*. I worried and thought a lot about feeding, and it was getting in the way of enjoying my family. I found dietitian and family therapist Ellyn Satter's work, and what I learned and applied about how to feed *felt right*. I was no longer anxious, and the more I saw my family thrive, the easier this new feeding style was.

I dug into the research about the medical and mental health issues related to my patients' struggles with food, eating, and weight. I was honored to join Ellyn Satter's clinical faculty for two years, rounding out my learning about relational feeding with interviews, research, and training on feeding disorders and therapies. Helping children grow up feeling good about food and their bodies is the best preventive medicine I can think of! It is gratifying to empower parents to bring their children from a place of fear (or preoccupation with food) to a healthy, joyful experience of food.

Over time, I saw more children with extreme picky eating. Almost universally, their parents were intensely involved and desperate for help. With an open mind, I've learned from pediatric dietitians, family therapists, speech therapists, occupational therapists, and psychologists. Most of all, I've learned to listen to and trust what devoted and caring parents share about what has and hasn't helped their families.

I (Jenny) am a speech-language pathologist (SLP) and since graduate school I have worked with children struggling to learn how to eat. I'm also the mom of three young children with vastly different feeding temperaments. Although I work daily with families with feeding issues, my experiences at home provide invaluable insights. While my first child always loved to eat and devoured sashimi at age four, my second child had about thirty to fifty accepted foods at the same age. His highly independent nature and emotional temperament definitely play a role in his selectivity. He reminds me daily that feeding is not so easy after all! The jury is still out on my toddler daughter.

Over a decade ago, I was working in an environment where applied behavioral analysis (or behavioral modification therapy) was the prescribed treatment method, and I found the strict rules required for that kind of therapy didn't sit well with me. The philosophy of "take a bite and you get to watch a video or play with this toy" wasn't working at home for many of the parents, and to me it felt completely unnatural to try to teach children to eat this way.

I explored the research and discovered strategies that worked better, eventually joining a university team. There, I developed a program that did feel good—for me and for the parents with whom I worked. I called it "STEPS," for "Supportive Treatment of Eating in PreschoolerS," and have since worked with hundreds of families within this framework of support, guidance, and skill building. Although STEPS focuses on children aged two to five, I frequently see newborns, and work with children up to age sixteen.

I've had the opportunity to work with occupational and physical therapists as well as dietitians, allowing me to see how sensory problems, motor delays, relationship blips, and combinations of these factors can start a child off on the wrong foot during early feeding. In my role as feeding supporter, I am privileged to help parents navigate their child's journey to food enjoyment. Over the years, I have learned that the ultimate goal for me and for the parents I work with is this: trusting the child, reading her cues, and helping her trust you. The rest is gravy!

Over the years, as we (Katja and Jenny) talked over some of our more challenging cases, we realized we offer similar guidance: establishing routine, uncovering counterproductive feeding practices, rehabilitating family meals, and reducing anxiety and power struggles, as well as brainstorming ways to address sensory and oral motor challenges.

We are both *committed to the principle that the trust and relationship between parent and child cannot be sacrificed for nutrition or growth goals.* As Black and Aboud (2011) put it, not feeding in a responsive way "has the potential to undermine the child's trust in an otherwise responsive parent."

The heart of this book is that parent-child partnership, and it's the cornerstone of the STEPS+, or *Supportive Treatment of Eating in PartnershipS,* approach. STEPS+ unites Jenny's more clinical oral motor and sensory support (with the parent as "therapist") with Katja's emphasis on the feeding relationship. Relational and therapeutic approaches to feeding challenges are best used together, with the child's response and comfort guiding the way: STEPS+ shows you how.

In building on and developing our own practice styles and strategies, we have incorporated aspects of the groundbreaking work of other researchers and clinicians. We are particularly grateful to Suzanne Evans Morris, Marsha Dunn Klein, Ellyn Satter, Debra Beckman, Catherine Shaker, and Irene Chatoor. With this book, we aim to share what we believe are the best and most helpful strategies available.

Becoming Your Child's Expert

You know your child best. You are your child's feeding expert—or at least that is what you will become. We will help you explore your child's temperament and reaction to change, and we will offer suggestions and clinically proven strategies to empower you to discover what does and does not work for your family. *We* trust *you.* We trust that by understanding challenges and using concrete strategies to work toward realistic goals, you will learn to feel competent and confident, and to understand where you or your family might benefit from additional support. Over time you will learn to trust yourself.

Overcoming feeding challenges can be a long process, and sometimes progress seems hard to recognize. Looking back on where you started can remind you of how far you have come. One of the most helpful tools in this process is a journal in which you record your frustrations, observations, and progress. Journaling may seem like just one more thing to do, but even if it's just a few pages in your kitchen drawer, your journal can prove invaluable. (One mom, frustrated by an apparent lack of progress, realized when reading back a few weeks that her son no longer cried for crackers first thing. Progress indeed!) Start with your journey so far, then write down a word or two every day (or pages). Note any positives (no crying; no tantrum; he passed a food at the table without making a face), or what happened when you tried a new routine or served carrots in circle-shaped coins instead of sticks. Note your and your child's attitude and feelings, not just her intake.

Parents often ask: "How long will it take?" Unfortunately, no one can predict. Some parents jump in and successfully change everything at once. Others need more support and move more slowly. Some children adapt quickly, eager for change, while others do better with a slower pace. Many parents are surprised at how quickly attitude improves and anxiety decreases—the basis for all other progress. We *can* predict that it will probably take longer than you'd like to see your child eating more of a variety of foods or in higher quantity. But we've also seen preschoolers with no apparent appetite, eating only a few foods, say, "I'm hungry," and taste new foods within days. We've seen tweens learn to like new foods within a few months. Typically, we see families make significant progress within three to twelve months (though for more severe issues it can take longer).

Along the way, you may slip into old habits and make "mistakes." This can slow the process, but these moments are opportunities to observe and learn. There will be triumphs and setbacks, and progress may look like steps forward and back rather than predictable, steady improvement. This is an expected (if confusing) part of the process. Be kind to yourself and your child, however this journey unfolds for you, and remember that change takes time. But it will be worth it.

CHAPTER 1

Understanding Typical Eating

There is incredible variability in the human experience, and all children are born with differences in temperament and more. However, a basic understanding of how children typically learn to eat helps you gauge how far off track your child might have wandered, and at what point. Moreover, understanding what's typical is rarely part of the training of the professionals you turn to for guidance, and it matters—consider the child whose major challenges were dismissed by her pediatrician, or the child with typical picky eating who was referred to intensive therapy that did more harm than good. Gaining a basic understanding is critical as you advocate for the best care for your child.

What surprises many parents is that typical eating is unpredictable, with children eating large amounts some days and little on others, and refusing favorite foods on a whim. Typical growth and development, as well as temperament and other factors, exist on a continuum. One child walks at ten months, another at thirteen—both are developing at a different pace within the normal range. Eating is no different.

Normal vs. Typical

We prefer the term "typical" to describe the most common patterns or time frames for the majority of children, understanding that there is a range. We are cautious about using the term "normal," as it can imply judgment, and each child's "normal" will differ, particularly with challenges. That is, a child's eating may be normal for her, but not typical. When a diagnosis is implied or needed, we may use "normal," acknowledging that the line between "normal" and "pathology" is rarely clear. Remember that if something is harming your child's emotional, physical, or social development or functioning, it is a problem for him and your family, regardless of terminology.

The continuum of typical eating is wide and varies across individuals (including children), families, and cultures. In this chapter, we'll explore this continuum as it pertains to how much children eat, how they grow, the development of physical skills involved in eating, and temperament.

Understanding Typical Intake

Young children don't eat the way we're told they should. They don't consume exact recommended portions, and what they eat won't look like the "MyPlate" chart at the doctor's office or stack up against a food pyramid or calorie chart. Most resources on feeding include portion size guidelines, increasing parents' anxiety if their child eats less (or wants more) than recommended.

We are glad that, increasingly, portion recommendations are listed as a starting place, with the caveat that the child may leave food on the plate or ask for more. As we explore in the next chapter, understanding the range of typical intake is critical: the harder we try to make children eat prescribed amounts, the more frustrated everyone becomes and the less well the children eat.

What and how much children eat varies greatly from meal to meal, day to day, and week to week. One dad said, "I can't accept that my son can go all afternoon on two bites of graham cracker." But he can! Consider these points:

- Young children may only eat one or two things at each meal or snack: for example, fruit one meal and pasta the next.

- Some children eat far more than recommended portions, while others eat less and still grow in a healthy way.

- Young children typically prefer carbohydrates (pasta, bread, sweets). This preference tends to diminish naturally as children mature.

- Intake varies based on energy and activity level. Illness, such as a cold, can decrease intake. Growth spurts can increase intake.

- Intake may decrease for a time as toddlers leave the rapid growth of infancy behind. Parents often find this confusing.

Pediatric dietitian Hydee Becker shared this encouraging assessment with us: "I have been looking at children's food logs for over fifteen years. Parents often report their child eating a few bites of this and drinking a few ounces of that, yet nutrition balances out over several days and the analysis usually looks fine."

Understanding Typical Growth

The biggest worry for parents usually relates to growth: small size, slow weight gain, or a child labeled as "underweight" on the growth charts or as "failure to thrive" (FTT). Yet *children who are small but growing in a steady way can be healthy.* The largest determinant of your child's adult height and weight is genetics. Consider your family history and growth patterns. One mom was surprised to see her own childhood growth chart starting out at the bottom of the curve and slowly increasing to average height and weight by high school.

Younger children tend to grow in "spurts," some of which happen over twenty-four hours with intervals of no growth for up to two months. Your son may wear size two pants for years, then need a new wardrobe seemingly overnight! This is why following growth over time is critical. Other important points about growth:

- Some healthy children move from higher to lower percentiles in the first two years. It isn't always cause for alarm.

- Growth that accelerates or slows is still probably healthy growth if the change is gradual and steady, and if your child is otherwise well and eventually settles at a relatively stable percentile, even at or below the "underweight" cutoff.

- Boys might be pressured more than girls to eat and be "big and strong."

Growth charts (see Figure 1.1) are often misinterpreted, even by doctors, with harmful consequences. They are not a report card or a standardized test of your parenting, where tenth percentile is worse than fiftieth. Tenth percentile may be right where your child should be. The percentiles only tell us how big or small a child is relative to a sampling of children the same age. Humans come in a variety of shapes and sizes; most people fall between the fifteenth and eighty-fifth percentiles, and some will naturally be smaller or larger.

Labels can also mislead. The labels "normal," "underweight," and "overweight" imply diagnostic certainty, while in fact, the cutoff percentiles for these categories are relatively arbitrary, differ by country, and have changed over the years. We see the label "failure to thrive"

(FTT) applied inconsistently—based on weight, or height-to-weight ratios ranging from the first to the tenth percentiles, or when children move downward on a growth chart (see Figure 1.2). We've also seen use of charts not corrected for prematurity, for those infants born early. Because the term is often incorrectly applied, if your child is labeled FTT, be sure to get a second opinion. Changes on the growth chart are important to consider, but it's not the whole picture. Looking at that big picture, one dad was empowered to say, "My son is *thriving*: happy, healthy, active, sleeping well. He's just small. If there's a problem with growth, let's call it that. My son is not 'failing' anything." Words matter.

Tracking a child's growth over time contributes to the overall picture of health and development. Since the labels and charts used to make sense of a child's growth measurements can confuse that picture, we recommend parents follow these tips to understand growth:

- Insist on accurate measurements, experienced staff, and the same clothing each time.

- Use charts corrected for prematurity.

- Plot your child's growth yourself. You may be the first to accurately plot her growth, uncovering a stable and healthy growth pattern (see "Helpful Resources" at http://www .newharbinger.com/31106 for an app to plot growth).

- Use weight-to-length ratios up to age three.

- Beyond age three, a combination of measurements is best (don't rely on BMI). Growth spurts are less frequent after this age, so a knowledgeable practitioner can help interpret growth.

The smooth growth curve you see at the doctor's office implies that healthy growth is smooth and continuous, when it is just as likely not. Children may grow in height very quickly, and then gain weight, so their weight-to-height ratio may look like a wavy line.

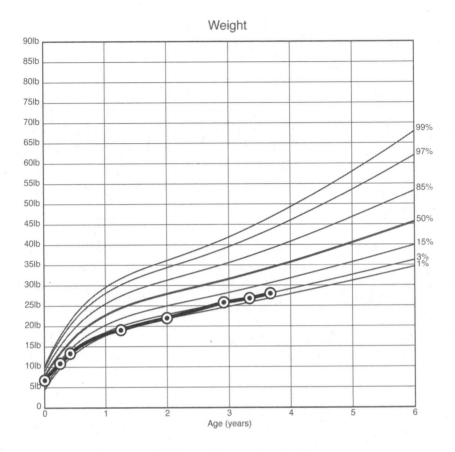

Figure 1.1. Low and Stable Growth

Figure 1.1 illustrates low and stable weight. If an evaluation of medical, feeding, and health behaviors doesn't indicate a concern, this is probably healthy growth. Continue behaviors that support health.

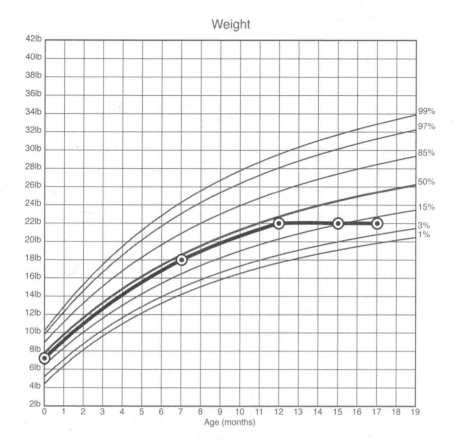

Figure 1.2. Growth Slowing

Figure 1.2 shows weight rapidly decreasing across percentiles; the child needs evaluation. A slow decline followed by leveling off of the growth trajectory also warrants evaluation, but may not be problematic.

Understanding the Mechanics of Learning to Eat

The process of learning to eat solids takes two to three years, typically beginning around six months of age when the child shows readiness, including sitting with little support and leaning toward or reaching for food. (Around age three, typically developing children eat somewhat like adults from an oral motor perspective.) The mechanics of learning to eat include increasing stability of the jaw and tongue and coordinating jaw, tongue, and cheek movements. Although we summarize it in a few sentences, learning to eat is complex—fully described in *Pre-Feeding Skills,* the 798-page reference book for parents and professionals by Suzanne Evans Morris and Marsha Dunn Klein (2000). And research continues to uncover new insights.

Still, eating well is more than either mechanics or trying a food ten times, as common feeding advice implies. First, children need a context—ideally, seeing caregivers enjoying eating. Then they get used to the look and smell by playing with the food as older infants, squishing and smearing it. (Think of those first-birthday cake frosting photos.) They may put food in their mouths and spit it out several times, or lick their fingers. They may love some foods (think carbs and sweets) the first time they try them, while others take many more exposures.

Typically developing kids can also refuse foods for no apparent reason. The child who happily ate eggs will pass on them for months (even years), then one morning reach for them again. Knowing this is normal reminds parents to keep those foods available, without pressure, until the child is ready to enjoy them again.

Normal Gagging

Virtually every child gags while learning to eat. The gag reflex protects the airway, keeping children from choking on things too big to swallow. If solids are introduced before the infant is ready, or foods don't match the child's skills, you may see frequent gagging. With more opportunities to eat lumpier and more challenging foods, the child learns that he has to mash and chew them before swallowing, and the gag disappears. The gag reflex's trigger point also moves from the front of the mouth to farther back as anatomy changes with growth. Chewing and mouthing nonfood objects also leads to a less sensitive trigger and less gagging.

Skills and experiences vary: one child may suck and gum teething biscuits while another chomps off huge chunks, gagging impressively every time. The chomper can skip biscuits and progress to lumpy foods.

Sensory Processing

Sensory processing refers to how humans experience input from the environment. We receive sound through our ears and light through our eyes; canals in our ears sense our body's position in the world; nerve endings on our fingertips and tongues and in our noses deliver information about touch, taste, and smell. This information is relayed to the brain, where it is integrated and compared to past experiences.

Sensory processing difficulties are often cited as *the* cause of most EPE. With sensory integration problems, sensory input can be interpreted as very intense or barely there. Foods with mixed textures can feel highly irritating and uncomfortable, while slippery or smooth foods that provide little input can be disorienting. Experiences that are neutral or pleasant for most people can feel overwhelming or painful for someone with sensory problems, contributing to a reluctance to eat.

But we all exist on a sensory continuum. Some of us chew gum or tap our feet to feel alert or calm. Some children may squeeze you too hard for comfort, grind their teeth, or hold their hands over their ears seeking sensory regulation. One child thrills at the hubbub of a state fair, while her sibling is overwhelmed by the lighting and noise at the local grocer.

The ability to synthesize sensory input and filter out what doesn't need attention are key factors in whether a child falls within the "normal" range of sensory processing. Consider Katja's nephew, a competent eater with traits commonly listed as criteria for a sensory disorder: he has reacted strongly to smells, refused mixed foods (typical of the toddler phase), and bitten his fingers and tongue while eating. He avoids autoflushing toilets and air hand dryers in public restrooms, despises tags in clothing, and startles at loud noises. He is happy and thriving with his way of experiencing the world and is growing more comfortable with sounds, clothing textures, and so on. If your child's sensory traits do not interfere with his overall happiness and development, you could choose to think of those traits simply as part of the spectrum of human experience.

Understanding Feeding Temperaments

You can think of your child's interest in and reactions to food as his *feeding temperament*—another continuum, from curious and willing to try new things to extremely cautious. How he approaches food will likely be similar to how he approaches life. We find that most children with EPE fall on the more wary side. A cautious temperament combined with sensory issues can make eating particularly hard. Also consider whether your child is strong-willed, wants to do things himself, or is anxious.

Many moms tell us their children ate differently *from birth*: one fed with gusto, while the other fell asleep and nursed on and off for hours. Acknowledging that children are born with unique feeding temperaments allows parents to let them be who they are when it comes to eating, without feeling the need to change them. Jenny sees different growth patterns and appetites with her two boys: one eats similar amounts at each meal while the other eats lots at breakfast and relatively little the rest of the day, with the occasional feast during a growth spurt. One was large (ninety-ninth percentile) from birth, while the other grew at around the fiftieth percentile from day one.

Food for Thought: The following statements help you understand your own feeding temperament and, in turn, how you might relate to your child's interest (or lack of interest) in food. Rate them on a scale of 1 ("strongly disagree") to 5 ("strongly agree"), with 3 being neutral:

I sometimes forget to eat.

I enjoy eating.

I feel antsy if I get hungry and don't have access to food.

I am not hungry for breakfast first thing.

When I plan my day, I always consider when and what I'm going to eat.

Understanding the role that temperament plays in your child's eating protects you from advice and meddling. For example, when a doctor or another parent swears that making a child take a "no-thank-you bite" of everything on her plate works, it may be that he or she has a more easygoing or adventurous child. Understanding temperament also helps parents grasp why one of their children struggles while the others don't, especially with no other diagnoses or obvious oral motor or sensory issues.

Understanding Development

While there is a typical range, children born prematurely or with developmental delays tend to take longer to learn to eat. One client had a baby who learned to walk at seventeen months, and her eating was also progressing about four to six months behind her peers. Expecting every child to develop in the same way sets you up for problems.

With typical development, gross motor skills (head and trunk control, sitting up) develop before fine motor skills (picking up a Cheerio between thumb and index finger); *oral motor skills are fine motor skills*. The rate of development of both fine and gross motor skills impacts eating. And while some children with a delay need help from formal feeding therapies, many who are progressing and otherwise doing well simply need support. Let's look at how developmental stages can impact feeding.

Infants: Transitioning to Solids and Self-Feeding

Typically, at around five or six months (adjusted age for preemies), infants show signs of readiness for solids: the ability to hold up their heads and torsos, open their mouths for the spoon, close their lips around the spoon, and not immediately push the food out with their tongues (the *tongue-thrust reflex*, which they're born with and which usually fades between four and six months of age).

Some parents spoon-feed purees while others skip spoons, allowing the older infant to pick up foods that she can suck on and mash with her gums (described in Tracey Murkett and Gill Rapley's 2010 book *Baby-Led Weaning*). Spoon-feeding is not by definition overfeeding or pressuring if the child invites the spoon (some babies even grab the spoon to direct it to their mouths) and enjoys the experience, and if you respond to and follow her cues.

Some babies enjoy being spoon-fed; others want to feed themselves. Other babies initially accept the spoon and then refuse it (usually at around eight to ten months). This is a common bump in the road, yet both of us have had calls from frantic parents whose older infants were labeled with an "oral aversion" because they "won't take the spoon anymore." We encourage these parents to give the child the spoon, or else to transition to soft finger foods, allowing the child more control, and often we hear back within days that the child is again eating happily.

Toddlers: Caution and Control

Toddlers and their parents can experience a perfect storm of challenges around feeding and eating. Even the most adventurous and confident eaters can go through a naturally picky phase from about fifteen months to around four years. During this cautious phase (characterized by *neophobia*, or fear of new things) they may become suspicious of even previously enjoyed foods, not want foods to touch on their plate, and pick out anything green.

Children say no as they go through the developmental task of becoming individuals—they may say no to putting on a jacket or brushing their teeth, or no to anything you want them to eat. In a bid for control, most will try to get parents to serve their favorites. In addition, growth and intake often slow, which is scary for parents of smaller children and can lead to parents only offering favorite foods. With all of these changes, this is a time when things often go wrong, but if parents know it's coming, with STEPS+ this stage doesn't have to derail feeding.

Preschoolers and Older Children: Competence and Relationship

Children aged around three to ten generally want to please parents, learn new tasks, and feel competent. As children reach the age of around seven to eight, many look for stronger relationships with peers, may have strong reactions to authority figures, and show increasing understanding of and concern for others. They become more aware of themselves and of how others perceive them. Although most enjoy their increasing independence and the responsibilities that come with it, children may experience guilt and shame when they don't do well. With feeding difficulties, they may desperately want to please you or "do well" at eating, and experience real distress when they are unable to do so.

Developing an understanding of your child's situation requires knowledge about the range of typical eating development in children; consideration of intake, growth, mechanics, temperament, and developmental stage deepen this understanding.

In the next chapter you'll build on your understanding of normal variation and delve into common eating challenges that can keep children from doing well. Even without getting into specific strategies to address challenges, this understanding can make a huge difference. One parent reported to us that learning what issues might factor in her son's picky eating helped her connect the dots and problem-solve creatively. As G.I. Joe put it, "Knowing is half the battle."

CHAPTER 2

Understanding Your Child's Challenges

In the introduction, we suggested that you'll learn to trust yourself and your child around food. That may feel impossible when you worry that she won't eat enough and hasn't progressed in months or years, and that things may even be getting worse. In this chapter you'll build on your understanding of development to explore feeding challenges and learn how extreme picky eating evolves. This knowledge will help you decide what you can let go of and what you can work on to support your child's eating and, above all, how to not make matters worse. Understanding your child and the challenges you both face is the work of these first chapters and the foundation for the steps ahead.

To recap, we define *extreme picky eating* (EPE) as not eating enough quantity or variety to support healthy emotional, physical, or social development; or eating patterns that are a significant source of conflict or worry. Here are some signs that your child may have more than typical picky eating:

Emotional

Is upset or cries often around food

Feels bad about his eating

Physical

> Has documented nutritional deficiencies
>
> Is falling off her own growth curve
>
> Has poor energy and/or frequent meltdowns when hungry

Social

> Can't go to sleepovers or social gatherings
>
> Isolates herself due to menu limitations
>
> Is teased by peers, or extreme attention is paid to her eating by adults (family, teachers)

"Children do well when they can" is a theme of *The Explosive Child* by Ross Greene (2010). If your child *can't* do well with eating right now, recognizing this and creating an environment where she *can* do well is the first step toward improving her relationship with food.

Feeding Challenges from Your Child's Point of View

Children with EPE are not just being naughty or willful (though they are at times more than capable of being so). Addressing feeding problems is not a matter of "breaking" your child or making her comply. Rather, *there is almost always an underlying reason that starts a child and his parents down the path of feeding difficulties.* Your struggles may have started in the neonatal intensive care unit, during the transition to self-feeding, or in the tricky toddler phase. Often, a definitive diagnosis or explanation for why your child struggles may not ever surface, despite extensive testing and evaluations. But since research shows that children with different initial feeding challenges develop similar presentations (Harris, Blissett, and Johnson 2000), you *can* help her even without a clear diagnosis.

Still, understanding (to whatever degree possible) the factors that contribute to your child's challenges and the dynamics at play can help you empathize with your child and be patient with the process. The STEPS+ approach can guide you, whether there are sensory issues, temperament considerations, or oral motor weaknesses. Here are the most common challenges, as seen from your child's point of view.

Medical Challenges: "It hurts! It doesn't feel good!"

Contributing medical issues must be ruled out or addressed. These might include allergies, reflux, eosinophilic esophagitis (painful allergy-related erosions of the esophagus), or severe constipation—basically anything that can cause pain or make a child feel poorly. As Harris and colleagues (2000) point out, "Pain and nausea, when associated with eating, is probably one of the best predictors of subsequent food refusal" (150). Young children can't identify what doesn't feel right, but they know it's difficult or painful, and their feeding behaviors are driven by avoiding negative feelings. Cardiorespiratory or muscular conditions that increase the effort necessary just to breathe, such as congenital heart defects, chronic lung disease, or muscular dystrophy, also impact feeding and often increase calorie needs.

The current criteria for diagnosing avoidant/restrictive food intake disorder (ARFID) say that you can't diagnose a feeding disorder when there is a medical illness. We think this is an oversimplification. Medical problems are often the root cause of a feeding problem *that persists* even after the medical issue has resolved. Interestingly, Harris and colleagues (2000) note that feeding problems that develop in children with medical conditions were essentially the same as those in children with no identified medical cause.

Oral Motor Challenges: "I can't."

Any physical issue that makes it hard to get food to the mouth, chew, breathe, swallow, or sit upright impacts eating. If it takes all of your child's energy and concentration to hold up her torso and head, she may not be able to eat long enough to achieve fullness. Anatomical problems like a cleft palate, malformations of the trachea or esophagus, dental issues, or even enlarged adenoids and tonsils can play a role. A frequently missed and easily corrected problem is tongue-tie, where a restrictive band of tissue holds the tongue to the floor of the mouth, affecting tongue motion and eating (including breastfeeding).

Proper jaw function is the foundation for oral motor skills, including coordinated tongue movement to transfer food, lip closure to keep food in, and tightening of the cheek muscles to keep food out of the cheeks. Jaw stability depends on balanced movement of facial and jaw muscles. Many children with oral motor difficulties lack coordinated chewing, tending to bite food toward the front of the mouth and not moving pieces requiring greater chewing force and precision to the back teeth. Take Mary, who was frustrated when sensory play therapies didn't address her son's chewing: "He's pushing food with his tongue between his teeth. He's four, and he chews like his ten-month-old sister. He wants to eat different foods, but he doesn't know what to do with food in his mouth."

Even subtle oral motor deficits can be a factor. Moving the tongue only in and out and up and down leaves children able to eat only soft, mashable foods; many get stuck at this level. Coordinated lateral (sideways) movement of the tongue is necessary for chewing harder foods and collecting food out of the cheeks and teeth to be swallowed. If your child can't chew with gums and early molars by about fifteen months (adjusting for prematurity) and progress has stalled, an evaluation with a qualified speech therapist can determine if there is a problem, and how to help (see chapter 8).

Sensory Challenges: "I don't like how this feels/tastes/looks/sounds. I'm uncomfortable."

Children with sensory integration challenges process sensory input differently, as reviewed in the last chapter. Brain imaging studies show visible differences in children with severe sensory processing disorder (SPD) compared with neurologically typical children (Owen et al. 2013). Tastes and textures can feel too intense, or awareness of food can be poor, leading to indifference or to "pocketing" (food stuck in the cheeks) because the child simply can't sense that the food is there. Some children with sensory challenges eat only smooth or crunchy foods with uniform texture. However, the tendency to reject mixed foods is also seen in typically developing children during the toddler phase.

Brain imaging also shows that taste and tactile processing differences are linked to eating difficulties. Visual processing has not yet been linked to food aversion, despite parental reports that children won't eat foods that *look* a certain way. Researchers theorize that this tendency is not caused by problems with visual perception and integration so much as the fact that the visible characteristics of the foods trigger fear based on past negative experiences (Farrow and Coulthard 2012).

While a sensory processing disorder presents a challenge, it doesn't mean a child is incapable of learning to expand her tastes and tolerate different sensory input. Alexa, mother of a child with severe sensory processing struggles, notes: "Amy is almost twelve, and in the last year we have seen incredible improvements in the variety she eats."

Many children with EPE eat foods of a variety of textures. If your child eats foods of different textures (say, yogurt, pretzels, and watermelon versus only purees), major sensory or oral motor problems are less likely to be present. That being said, every child has sensory preferences, just like adults. And all foods are new at first, with some ending up legitimately disliked for whatever reason. You won't necessarily know what those are yet for your child, and you might not know for some time. (As adults, both of us—Katja and Jenny—want to like olives but we can't get there!)

Some examples of sensory preferences include:

Taste/Smell

Likes only bland or strong flavors

Prefers the same few flavors

Turned off by strong smells

Visual

Doesn't like bright lights

Finds patterns distracting

Only eats from certain packaging or brands

Tactile

Wants hands wiped of any mess, or isn't aware of food on face or hands

Doesn't like mixed textures or prefers crunchy textures

Distracted by feet dangling during meals

Prefers food at certain temperatures

Auditory

Reacts to noise more than peers do

Prefers music or steady background noise

Exhibits stress long after an unexpected noise has stopped

Responding to your child's sensory preferences should guide your daily choices; for example, you might need to avoid loud and crowded restaurants, be sure his chair has a stable footrest, or add crunch to foods (see chapter 7).

Food for Thought: List foods you didn't like as a child, and describe *why*. Has your list changed since then? Describe characteristics of foods you do and don't like (soft; chewy; wet; fruits with skins or seeds).

Although SPD is getting more research and attention, it remains controversial for many practitioners. Sensory challenges often exist with other disorders, including attention deficit disorder and anxiety, which should be ruled out as part of a thorough evaluation. In addition, it can be tricky to know where to draw the line on a sensory continuum between a normal variant and a disorder. Many children grow out of their sensitivities, and parents also have valid concerns about labels. Without adequate high-quality research to guide decisions about SPD treatments at this time, trust your gut as to whether or not to pursue sensory therapies, therapies to address behavioral challenges or anxiety, or a combination.

Sensory Processing Problems and Hunger and Fullness Cues

Some professionals say that children with SPD or sensory problems can't sense hunger and fullness cues (like their stomachs stretching). We think this makes quite a leap. Rather, we would say that learning to tune in to those cues is a skill; and while some children have a lower awareness of appetite cues—meaning it may be harder to tune in to those sensations—the vast majority of children, even those with GI or sensory issues, can learn to eat an appropriate amount based on cues of hunger, fullness, and appetite. This is known as *self-regulation*, and with the supportive feeding described in this book, it can be achieved. In fact, if a child has less ability to sense cues, it's even more important to keep the background noise—anxiety, pressure, fear, or stress—to a minimum so the child can tune in to the cues.

Regulating intake is far more complex than just sensing input from the stomach; it encompasses complex hormonal feedback loops and blood-sugar levels, calorie regulation, and more (Sanger, Hellstrom, and Naslund 2010). For most of the children we've seen with sensory problems and apparent lack of appetite, the sensory piece was *not* the main issue. Challenges most often included extreme anxiety, pressure or conflict around feeding, distraction, or grazing. And almost always, *with opportunity and support*, appetite and eating abilities improved.

Sensory Seekers Crave Input

Sensory seeking is a subset of sensory processing problems. Seekers seem to be less aware of sensory input—they are hyposensitive rather than hypersensitive. They may bite their tongues or fingers often, or drool and eat with their mouths open. Some sensory seekers seem completely unaware of flavor, happily eating foul-tasting foods (like skunk-flavored jellybeans). More commonly, sensory seekers look for input through crunchy, sour, or spicy foods, extreme temperatures, or carbonated drinks. Beyond food, they might love getting messy, like strong hugs, or crash their bikes repeatedly. Adding crunchy pretzel pieces to a sandwich or cinnamon to chilled applesauce provides the input these children seek out, which can help sensory seekers maintain attention at meals. (More ideas in chapter 8.)

To further complicate things, we've seen children with seeking *and* avoiding behaviors: for example, avoiding varied textures but craving intense spice; or recoiling from loud noises while seeking intense physical stimuli.

Temperament and Mood: "I don't want to! I want to do it my way."

Many of our clients describe their children similarly: highly verbal and intelligent; having a strong desire to figure things out in their own time and their own way; easily upset and frustrated; and feeling and expressing intense emotions. Many neurologically typical children with EPE exhibit an independent nature (determined and not wanting to lose), or are very tuned in to a parent's agenda and pressure, resulting in increased anxiety. Food refusal has been linked to temperament traits including shyness, emotionality, and irritability. We also note that many of our clients' children have struggled with toilet training or constipation. We suspect that is no coincidence—as the expression goes, "There are three things you can't make a child do: eat, poop, and sleep."

Jenny discovered that any efforts to encourage her younger son to try something resulted in tears and less eating of even favorite foods. Although he no longer eats many foods he once did, he started eating peanut butter on bread again after a year of refusing, added back tomatoes, and learned to enjoy all colors of bell peppers after an afternoon of cooking with his mom. This is also the child who puts everyone's shoes away, taught himself to read at four, and gets wildly upset when told he's wrong. Sound familiar?

Negative Experiences: "I'm scared _____ will happen again."

Regulation of appetite, hunger, and intake involves a complex interplay of messages to the brain from various systems, with many ways the process can go wrong. If, in the past, acting on his desire to eat—his appetite—has resulted in an uncomfortable or scary sensation, a child's appetite may decrease. Aversive experiences can happen in typically eating children; for example, a choking episode can trigger a fear of choking to the point where a child stops eating and drops weight quickly.

Similarly, a child who has experienced coercive or forced feeding may develop an extreme fear that exacerbates initial challenges. One mom tearfully described how she put her son in a headlock to get the first bite in during a therapy protocol meal in his highchair: he was crying, his mom was crying, and from then on he screamed every time he saw the highchair. The highchair, eating, and appetite were now linked in his mind with a traumatic experience. Other aversive experiences include aspiration (food in airways or lungs) or vomiting.

Negative experiences can result in a child who may experience hunger, but whose appetite is effectively turned off.

> **Food for Thought:** Think back to the last time you had a stomach flu or food poisoning—did you want to eat? Were there foods you avoided after becoming well again? (This is an example of *aversive conditioning*.)

If your child suddenly stops eating or has major changes involving intake, food-related fears, or obsessive-compulsive thinking, then the (relatively new) diagnosis of pediatric acute neuropsychiatric syndrome (PANS) should be considered—though your doctor may not have heard of it. PANS is a rapid-onset brain-based illness occasionally triggered by infection. Considering or ruling out PANS, any underlying medical condition, an eating disorder, or an aversive experience is critical.

The Sensorimotor Connection

Some children have more than one challenge. Williams and colleagues suggest that "in childhood feeding problems it is difficult, if not impossible, to separate behavior from biology" (2009, 132). Everything gets mixed together. Infants who don't mouth objects due to sensory problems are less likely to develop refined oral motor skills. If Jenny had a dollar for each parent seeking treatment who said her child never mouthed objects an as infant, she would be rich!

Conversely, oral motor problems can lead to sensory issues. When a child is born with oral motor weakness (for example, a child with Down syndrome and low muscle tone), the muscles in the cheeks, lips, and jaw don't function appropriately, so the nerve endings aren't properly activated. The "sensory-motor loop," as Debra Beckman calls it in her workshops, is effectively broken. The sensory and motor systems go hand in hand: if the sensory system doesn't alert the motor system that it's time to chew, small pieces of food may slip back toward the child's throat before he's ready to swallow. He may overstuff his mouth seeking sensory input, or gag or vomit frequently, which feels bad and lowers appetite. Add a child's cautious temperament or desire to do it his way, as well as a parent's reactions and frustrations, and you can see how hard it is to tease out causative factors.

> **Food for Thought:** To illustrate the sensorimotor loop, think about the last time a dentist numbed your mouth. What happened when you tried to eat, drink, or talk?

Misunderstandings and Feeding Problems

Sometimes a child has EPE without oral motor issues, developmental delays, or sensory problems. You might only recognize the temperament piece in your child. In such cases, we often find that a misguided concern about weight or delayed feeding skills was misinterpreted, leading to worry and inappropriate intervention. This matters because when parents are advised to feed in ways that are developmentally inappropriate or invite pressure, *they can cause a feeding problem where none, or only minor blips, existed.*

Misunderstanding of Developmental Diversity

A common example of inappropriate concern and intervention involves the ex-preemie who has a hard time starting solids at six months. Many doctors fail to account for the number of weeks or months that a child was premature and adjust feeding expectations accordingly. Standard practice for premature infants is to adjust developmental expectations until they are between two and two-and-a-half years old, when most catch up with peers.

If your former preemie's pediatrician recommended starting solids at four or six months, you may have struggled to keep food in his mouth, growing increasingly frustrated. Maybe you even began to worry and exert pressure. One mom was chastised by her doctor for not starting her nine-month-old (six-and-a-half months, adjusted) twins on Cheerios, so she tried it and ended up with gagging, unhappy babies. Misguided concern led to inappropriate recommendations, relying on *chronological* rather than *developmental age.*

Misguided Worries About Growth

Misguided concern about weight often leads clinicians to recommend feeding practices that can cause or worsen feeding problems. Most typically this occurs with a premature baby or smaller than average child. For example, a baby woken with great effort every thirty minutes to breastfeed in order to increase her weight or her mother's milk supply will likely have trouble with her developmental task of homeostasis, or state regulation, which involves learning her body's rhythms of sleep, hunger, and fullness. This can lead to what Irene Chatoor (2009) calls "feeding disorder of state regulation," where the infant is unable to successfully integrate and regulate cycles of sleep and hunger.

After being told, "Do whatever you have to do to get those ounces in," some parents may syringe breast milk or formula into the baby's mouth too quickly, or repeatedly reintroduce a bottle when the baby is upset, or hold the baby's head in place to get in a few more drops. These desperate efforts can lead to gagging and negative experiences—the baby learns that eating is scary. When infants struggle with early feeding, it sets them up for further difficulties.

Mistaking Gagging for Choking

Occasionally, from fear of choking, parents provide only smooth, thin foods that are easily swallowed long after the infant is ready for more challenging foods, and the infant misses out on the sensorimotor experiences that improve eating skills. When parents first see gagging, they often assume the child 1) is choking; 2) doesn't like the food; or 3) is uncomfortable. The child usually swallows after gagging and moves on to the next bite. But if the parent gets upset, the child may take cues from the parent that what happened was scary.

Gagging, as explained in chapter 1, is a normal response when the infant is learning to eat more textured food. Choking, by contrast, happens when food moves into the windpipe so the child can't breathe. Gagging is usually over in two to five seconds; the child continues to cough or make noises but isn't in distress. With choking, there is no sound, the child's color changes, and he appears more distressed. Every parent should have CPR training to learn to differentiate gagging and choking, as well as how to respond to the latter.

Diagnostic Considerations

As you are learning, feeding problems are incredibly complex issues not easily reduced to a list of symptoms or clearcut diagnoses. Many challenges are variations of normal eating stages or fall on a spectrum from typical to extreme picky eating; where to draw the line is not always clear. In order to consider the implications of a diagnosis, we'll explore factors influencing diagnosis and treatment.

Many definitions of "picky" versus "problem eating" use checklists or cutoffs based on the number of foods a child eats. This is problematic, since most parents give up offering a new food after very few tries. Understandably, parents worried about poor weight gain may offer only foods the child will reliably eat, or depend on supplement drinks "to get some calories in." Diagnosis is tricky, particularly when diagnostic criteria are influenced by the way a child has been fed.

For example, take a child who panics around oatmeal. This negative reaction is commonly used as a diagnostic criterion for sensory-based food aversion. Is this panic due to the sensory properties of the oatmeal, as the diagnosis suggests, or might it be the child's fear that she will be pressured to put the oatmeal in or near her mouth, as she has been for months? We've both had calls from incredulous parents explaining how a child who previously screamed at the sight of oatmeal now sits calmly while the parent or nanny eats it *right next to her.* This dramatic change occurred after only a few days of reassuring the child that *she* decides when and how to interact with food and will no longer be pressured.

It is critical to understand that every challenge, whether medical, sensory, or behavioral, happens within the context of the feeding relationship. If you define your child's issues solely by the medical or developmental challenge, as diagnoses imply you should, it is easy to focus on that one issue. For example, if the initial problem was reflux, then fixing the reflux should solve the problem, much like replacing a faulty carburetor in an old car that won't run. Alas, if there have been months of pain, fear, and conflict around feeding, you might fix that carburetor, but the car still won't run. (Ideally reflux is discovered and addressed early and you have support to avoid further problems.)

Reimbursement Impacts Diagnosis

In the United States, the diagnosis determines if your child's health insurance (whether private or government assistance) will pay for intervention, or if she receives services at school and how extensively. Parents may feel the need to seek, and clinicians to give, a particular diagnosis simply so that the child gets help. This may be necessary, but it's not ideal. Many sensory-based therapies, for example, are not currently covered by insurance, since there are few agreed-upon diagnoses and standard treatments. Parents and therapists have told us that for many insurance companies, a doctor's diagnosis of a "feeding disorder" clears the way for all therapies to be paid for. This is a strong incentive to diagnose a feeding disorder when something else may be going on.

With the increase in private therapy centers and reimbursement in the thousands of dollars for feeding therapies, there may also be incentive to recommend services for children who may not need them. Some centers operate with questionable ethics around the acceptance and continuance of patients in therapy. For example, a child may meet all of his goals, but new goals are added to keep him in therapy; or an expanded inpatient capacity means increased recommendations for inpatient therapy even when a less intensive approach may suffice. You should carefully consider any recommendation for inpatient treatment for a medically stable child. Inpatient stays are highly disruptive for families and can further traumatize children. Seek a second opinion, and ask to speak with parents who have been through the program.

Increasingly, therapies that we believe are unwarranted and potentially harmful are marketed to parents of children with typical picky eating. With about one-third of parents experiencing some picky eating, this is an enticing market for providers. In general, if things are going pretty well with feeding and you feel good about your progress, *don't let someone talk you into a diagnosis or therapy.*

Feeding Disorders vs. Eating Disorders

Colleagues working in the field of eating disorders tell us that children who have "failed" treatment for EPE are increasingly referred to eating disorder centers. Most of these professionals share that they did not train in nor are they familiar with how children learn to eat and what can go wrong. This matters because understanding a child's history and development around eating is critical to proper treatment. For example, new-onset anorexia at age nine requires different treatment than a food aversion going back to infancy.

Eating disorders are complex neuropsychiatric (brain-based) illnesses with genetic and environmental components, characterized by abnormal eating and distorted thinking about body image, that threaten a child's well-being and survival. Eating disorders occur at a range of weights, in boys and girls, and in every ethnic and socioeconomic group. The steps in this book support youth struggling with eating, but they are *not* substitutes for treatment for children with eating disorders.

Red flags for eating disorders include talk about wanting to lose weight or comments about preferring to be thin (body-image dissatisfaction); dieting; preoccupation with healthy eating or calories; or excessive exercise. Mood disorders like anxiety and depression are associated with eating disorders. Children with feeding disorders appear to be at increased risk of developing an eating disorder for reasons not yet fully understood (Kotler et al. 2011). Addressing feeding struggles may prevent the problem from developing into an ongoing eating disorder. *If you are at all concerned about the possibility that your child has an eating disorder, talk with your child's doctor.* Eating disorders require specialist diagnosis and treatment. For information, visit the National Eating Disorder Association's website (http://www.nationaleatingdisorders.org).

This chapter has asked you to consider your child's challenges and experiences so that you can understand how her efforts to avoid certain foods and situations help her feel comfortable, safe, and in control. If your child has had negative, painful, or forced feeding experiences, her "abnormal" eating behaviors are adaptations that protect her from further distress. The next chapter delves into how your responses to your child's challenges can contribute to her difficulties, and offers practical advice for changing your own behavior and your patterns of interaction with your child for the better.

CHAPTER 3

Understanding Your Role

You may have heard that "90 percent of feeding challenges are sensory" or that "It's all how Mom feeds" or "It's purely behavioral." But it's rarely so simple. So far, we've explored feeding challenges and factors that contribute to feeding problems, as well as how focusing on any one aspect of your child's eating situation means you may miss ways to help her. While you have limited or no control over some of your child's challenges, you do have control over your part in the feeding relationship. Your part includes how and when you offer food; the atmosphere you create and the expectations you hold; the words you say to your child; and what, if any, kinds of therapy you seek out. Whatever your child's challenges are, how you respond is crucial, and it's something you can change if you need to.

This chapter will explore how a worry-fueled response to initial feeding challenges and poor support combine to influence a child's eating. Pressuring children to eat results in anxiety or power struggles, and it almost always backfires. We understand that this may be a difficult chapter to get through. It's hard for parents to think that what they have done may have contributed to the problem, but remember that a sign of good parenting is asking for and finding help. In our experience, parents know when things aren't working and appreciate being taught to recognize and change counterproductive practices. Hang in there!

Understanding the Worry Cycle of Feeding

The *worry cycle* (see Figure 3.1) is a way for parents and childcare providers to visualize the dynamics at play in a feeding relationship that has gone awry. Our clients describe feeling like they are in a "black hole" or are "circling the drain" when stuck in this cycle. In the last two chapters we've covered feeding challenges that can begin the cycle. Here we'll explore what parents worry about and how fear-driven responses to the child's initial challenges drive the child's resistance.

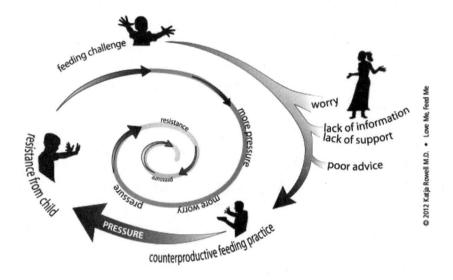

Figure 3.1. The Worry Cycle

Most parents of children with EPE worry about growth and nutrition. While some of these fears are founded, there may also be *perceived* challenges where none, or only relatively minor ones, exist. Consider this example. After a workshop, a mother of a twelve-month-old said: "I serve chicken nuggets every night because he'll eat them and he needs more protein." After a brief discussion, it was clear he was getting more than enough protein even without the nuggets. Two things were happening: 1) Mom was overestimating his protein needs, and 2) she was limiting his opportunities to learn to like other protein sources. He was not unusually selective, and had no delays or special needs. Out of an unfounded worry about nutrition (protein), Mom served only his favorites, increasing the odds he would refuse other protein sources and demand chicken nuggets.

Food for Thought: Have you started that journal yet? What nutrition or other worries can you write down off the top of your head? The following pages may spark some recognition of worries that drive your worry cycle.

In reality, nutrition is rarely an urgent matter. We all know adults who eat nowhere close to the dietary recommendations and are healthy and happy. In developed countries, actual deficiencies of most nutrients are relatively rare, thanks to fortified and enriched foods. Pushing "nutritious" foods on your child can, however, lead to power struggles—a setup for worse nutrition now *and* in the future. As Skye Van Zetten, mom of a child with EPE, wrote on her *Mealtime Hostage* blog, "Trying to make my son eat certain foods and get him to gain weight just made him not eat—at all."

It would be wonderful if every child devoured kale and blueberries, fish and avocado (and if every parent had access to and could afford these foods), but in real life, things are a bit more...interesting. It's not that nutrition isn't important, but including your child's "safe" (even less nutritious) foods will help you achieve your goal of improved variety and nutrition over time (more on supporting nutrition in chapter 7). Variety, rather than avoidance, is the key to good nutrition, which is why we aim for long-term development of the best possible food-acceptance skills. (Remember that variety differs from person to person, and that even adults who are relatively selective eaters usually meet their nutritional needs.)

Our goal in this section is to reassure you regarding some of the most common nutrition concerns, such as too much of some foods, too little of others, and food allergies. Hydee Becker, a pediatric dietitian with more than fifteen years' experience (including at a hospital feeding clinic), has contributed her insights throughout this section.

Worry About Deficiencies

If you worry about your child's nutrition, particularly perceived deficiencies, consider getting a detailed intake analysis. Ideally, this involves tracking what you offer, as well as when and how much your child eats, for seven days, including two weekend days. A registered dietitian can use this record to analyze your child's intake of calorie-providing macronutrients (fat, carbohydrates, and protein) and micronutrients (vitamins and minerals). (See the online Resources at http://www.newharbinger.com/31106 for intake analysis instructions and a template.) You may learn that your child is doing better than you think; if not, you'll have the information you need to address any shortfalls.

Not Enough Protein?

Protein is the most common macronutrient parents worry about. "He has to have protein at breakfast!" is a common refrain. Pediatric dietitian Hydee Becker says that protein is "almost never" low, even for children with EPE. Parents commonly overestimate how much protein children need. For example, a thirty-nine-pound preschooler meets his daily protein needs with one cup of cow's milk or soy beverage, two tablespoons of peanut butter, and two slices of bread (or alternatively, one 150-gram container of Greek yogurt and four chicken nuggets).

Not Enough Vegetables?

Parents often wish their children ate more vegetables. A quality multivitamin and mineral supplement provides needed micronutrients while you wait for your child's eating to improve. Fruits have many of the same nutrients as vegetables, as well as fiber (often low for children with EPE), which helps with bowel movements (BMs). If your child likes some fruits, serve those often and branch out with fruits first. Also, if you think of fruits and vegetables as a single group, you might find your child is doing better than you thought.

Chronic constipation often fuels worry about fruit and vegetable intake. Low fiber and fluid intake contribute to chronic constipation, but increasing fiber and fluids alone rarely solves the problem. Once there is significant constipation for weeks or months, the colon stretches, and it takes up to six months for the colon to return to proper shape and function. Chronic constipation can lead to decreased appetite, abdominal cramping and even vomiting—not to mention pain with BMs, triggering a natural reflex to withhold BMs. Over time, it's hard for a constipated child to recognize what his body is telling him (sound familiar?). Parents may encourage with, "Let it out, you will feel better," but the child simply can't comply.

Adding probiotics (beneficial bacteria) via food, drinks, or supplements can help promote a healthy gut, and it can't hurt as long as there aren't battles about getting them in. While you're working to optimize intake of liquids, fruits, and vegetables without pressure (the subject of chapter 7), a fiber supplement or intervention like MiraLAX (undetectable when dissolved in liquids) can help your child have daily, soft, pain-free BMs. Parents often stop stool softeners or laxatives too soon. Discuss the details with your doctor, but know that it may take several months for your child to learn to respond to her body's cues.

Not Enough Calcium?

Calcium, important for bone strength, is obtained mainly through dairy. If your child does not like dairy products or is allergic to dairy protein, his calcium needs can be met through calcium-fortified soy milk. If neither dairy nor soy foods are a regular part of your child's diet, look for other calcium-fortified foods such as orange juice. Ask your child's doctor or dietitian about calcium-rich foods or supplements while your child builds his food-acceptance skills. A multivitamin should help bolster vitamin D (which aids calcium absorption), especially in northern climates where there is less sunlight to stimulate the body's own vitamin D production.

What About Iron?

Iron isn't on most parents' radar, but for children with EPE, it can be difficult to get enough. Low iron can lead to poor appetite and delayed growth, and it may also lead to behavioral and neurodevelopmental changes and sleep disturbances. A simple finger-stick test screens for low iron and is the only blood test we recommend for all children with EPE. If her iron is low, your child may need more lab work, and she'll need supplements. Ask your doctor for dose, preparation, and follow-up. If iron levels remain low with adequate supplementation, it can indicate an underlying problem, such as food intolerance.

Other tests are at your doctor's or dietitian's discretion. Rarely, severe malnutrition or nutrient deficiencies (such as iron and zinc) can themselves dampen appetite—a vicious cycle. Better safe than sorry if there is any concern.

Worry About Excess

We believe that worry about specific "bad" foods or nutrients can do more harm than the foods themselves. Here we'll address sugar and salt; research on both is contradictory, and you'll find that some widely accepted "facts" and recommendations may not be so clear-cut.

Sugar

Sugar is the macronutrient currently blamed for society's health and nutrition woes, as fat was before it. While there is evidence that unbalanced intake of refined carbohydrates, including sugar (often added to processed foods to replace fat), can contribute to chronic health problems, blaming or demonizing one macronutrient or food doesn't support good feeding or nutrition.

We do not believe sugar is "toxic" or "addictive" per se, and a review of the research concluded, "There is no support from the human literature for the hypothesis that sucrose may be physically addictive or that addiction to sugar plays a role in eating disorders" (Benton 2010). Sugar is also often blamed for poor behavior. While studies haven't proven that sugar causes hyperactivity or behavior problems, if a child eats only sugar or refined carbohydrates, the blood-sugar spike and *following crash* may contribute to poor behavior. In addition, the *belief* that sugar causes children to misbehave can become self-fulfilling. Think of the times a child is told sugar makes him hyper, or is given a "treat" at school on an empty stomach, with lots of excitement and warnings about not getting out of control with all the *sugar*…

Almost universally, children like sweet tastes. Breast milk is naturally sweet, and in evolutionary terms, sweetness helps humans identify energy-rich foods, whereas bitterness may indicate toxins. A study by Coldwell, Oswald, and Reed in 2010 showed that children may outgrow their preference for markedly sweeter tastes during adolescence, around the time they stop growing. This suggests that the biological drive for growth is part of the reason for children's preference for sweetness and that children outgrow their taste for supersweet foods.

If you worry about sugar intake, here are some tips:

- When offering high-sugar foods, also offer protein, fat, and a fiber source. Pour a glass of milk or soy beverage, or serve with whole-grain crackers, cheese, or fruit and peanut butter.

- Consider candy or sweets containing fat and protein: Snickers bars, for example, with nuts and chocolate; or peanut M&Ms; or cookies with butter and whole-wheat pastry flour or oats.

- Remember that a little sweetness can *help* children branch out (see chapter 8).

If you're worried about your child getting enough calories, calming her food anxieties, or increasing the variety of her diet, try putting aside the sugar worry for the time being. Applying pressure or even avoiding fruit because of sugar fears means variety and nutrition suffer and anxiety goes up. As pediatric dietitian Hydee Becker says about sugars, "The benefit of added calories for growth is worth added sugar." We would also encourage you to set aside fears of high fructose corn syrup as well, which is almost identical to table sugar in makeup.

Salt

Don't worry about salt unless your child has a condition where salt matters, like kidney or heart disease. Processed foods tend to be high in salt, but even that doesn't worry us. In addition, when you stop trying to limit salt, your child may become less interested in it. There is no research support for limiting salt in healthy children, and it's controversial even for adults. Enjoy the relief that this is a battle you don't have to fight.

Worry About Allergies or Sensitivities

Parents faced with any number of diagnoses or developmental challenges will find online "cures" consisting of specialized or highly restrictive diets. (Be wary of unscrupulous companies and practitioners who prey on fear to sell pricy or questionably useful supplements.) Many overwhelmed parents can't handle one more regimen, and elimination diets are neither easy nor to be taken lightly.

Some kids are sensitive to the protein gluten (found in wheat, rye, barley, and sometimes oats), and this causes constipation, diarrhea, abdominal discomfort, or poor nutrient absorption. Others are sensitive only to wheat. Celiac disease, an autoimmune disease that tends to run in families, requires total elimination of gluten.

Many parents believe that eliminating one or more foods or food groups (meat, gluten, dairy, and so on) is the answer to various health concerns. In the absence of a true allergy or sensitivity, however, enforcing these restrictions can put an enormous burden on families, without clear benefit. If you are thinking about removing food groups from your child's diet, it is *essential* to work with a gastroenterologist, allergist, or dietitian specializing in food sensitivities. Talk with your health professional about the possibility of food sensitivities, true allergies, or other medical conditions including celiac disease.

While many parents would be thrilled if their child ate Cheetos, others serve only whole foods, or strictly avoid food dyes or additives. Some parents find that their children are sensitive to certain food dyes, and research (mostly small studies on children with attention deficit disorder) suggests that some children do react to certain dyes—often when they're at relatively high doses. Major food brands are listening to consumers and providing more options free from artificial dyes, sweeteners, and preservatives. Local co-ops and stores like Whole Foods and Trader Joe's stock foods free from these additives, and other large supermarket chains are following suit. If your child does better without artificial food dyes or preservatives and avoiding them isn't disrupting feeding, go ahead and eliminate them; but if you don't notice a difference, it may not be worth the additional effort and conflict.

Remember that *anxiety* about additives can be toxic. One mom of a preschooler with severe food anxieties shared how she ran across the kitchen and snatched a cracker out of her toddler's hand because it had processed flour and oil. Looking back, she wonders if this incident, and others like it, contributed to her son's fear of food.

Cochrane research review committees (impartial teams of research experts addressing specific clinical questions) were unable to find high-quality evidence that elimination diets (or various supplementation regimens) made a difference in a reproducible way for children with autism (Millward et al. 2008). More thorough and well-designed research is needed, but remember that your child is your best evidence. Although some families that follow elimination diets see improvement, just as many see no change. Chapter 8 briefly addresses elimination diets.

Shelve the Worries for Now

Nutrition worries lead to power struggles, and pressure tactics impede progress. Particularly with nutrition, *aiming for perfect is the enemy of good*. Skye Van Zetten (2013), the *Mealtime Hostage* blogger, advises, "Ignore the constant rhetoric about how many servings of something you should be eating, and how fat, sugar, salt, and well… food is bad for you. Seriously, turn all of it off. Sure, I would love to see my son eating a balanced diet from all four food groups, but he isn't at that level of eating competence yet. Right now, TJ is experimenting with food that tastes good—a huge improvement from the child who was too anxious to join us at the table a year ago."

In this book we don't recommend what to serve (or not) other than to offer suggestions toward variety, menu planning tips, and skill building, on the premise that *no food should be off limits to a child with EPE unless medically indicated*. Nutrition is important, but this book is about the *how* of feeding. *What* you serve is always up to you, and there are myriad religious, cultural, time, and financial considerations, in addition to your family's preferences and foods your child will eat. We reject shaming, or labeling foods as "good" or "bad" in general, knowing that parents who want to feed the "right" foods feel terribly guilty when their children eat what others call junk. Working on *how* you feed and how your child feels about food will lead to better nutrition and health over time, while pressure to reach nutrition goals mostly backfires.

Why So Worried? Selling Fear and Bad Advice

We want to give our children the best, and we often feel guilty when that doesn't seem to work out. "Mommy guilt" is a phenomenon that marketers help create and promote. Companies successfully use fear and guilt to sell moms special bottles or baby-food makers, apps to track their child's intake, expensive eco-friendly items, supplements, and organic squeezie pouches. Why wouldn't they?

One worried mom reached out to Katja after reading online that the protein in her meat lasagna could damage her toddler's kidneys. With a healthy child, this is impossible, but every worry, question, or doubt is confirmed and amplified in our era of instant and constant information—and it undermines healthy feeding. This is one of many differences in parenting today compared to previous generations. Your parents and grandparents didn't read about DHA and brain development, worry about antioxidants, or suffer constant bombardment with media stories about nutrition and obesity as parents are today.

Today's parents are also raising children in a different economic reality from a generation or two ago. According to the USDA, at the time of writing, one in five children lives in a food-insecure home (meaning they have unreliable access to enough food). If you struggle to get enough food, or are concerned about spending money on foods your child is not likely to eat, we will address this in later chapters. We recognize the additional burden that financial worries and securing food assistance places on families struggling with feeding.

As we continue along the worry cycle, we move to the anxious parent with little support and plenty of poor advice—whether it's from the auntie who tells you to start solids with your three-day-old or the cousin advising you to "starve out" your "spoiled" girl. Books and other would-be reputable sources also offer poor recommendations. Consider an infant feeding web page from a well-known U.S. hospital system that advised *only* feeding with a spoon, since the infant "must" learn to eat from the spoon. Not only is there no evidence to support this statement, but what happens if he doesn't want the spoon? This advice sets up power struggles.

Most upsetting is when doctors, the people parents turn to for help, give some of the worst advice. Parents often ask, "Why doesn't our child's doctor know this?" Doctors don't know what they don't know. Their training is wide, but for most it doesn't include even basic information about feeding, growth, and nutrition. It's unclear why something that clinicians deal with daily—one in three parents asks the child's doctor for feeding help—gets little (if any) consideration in medical training. Jenny pushed for and provides a one-hour feeding training to pediatric residents from the local children's hospital, but that's all they get! Even some feeding therapy providers give less than helpful suggestions. Generally, if what you are told to do increases conflict, anxiety, or gagging and doesn't support family meals or routine, it is poor advice.

Parents also tell us that, in addition to giving poor advice, professionals often ignore their concerns. When a third child is very different from the first two and isn't progressing with eating, being told "He'll grow out of it" or "Stop worrying; make him what he likes" is less than helpful. Since the old definitions of feeding problems relied on weight loss, parents were told not to worry as long as the child was growing. One father's tween son only ate plain cheese quesadillas for six years. Every year, as the boy grew in the normal range, Dad's concerns and requests for help were ignored. Knowing that your child's doctor didn't know the difference between typical picky eating and more complex concerns makes the bad advice and lack of guidance understandable, if not forgivable.

And many children *do* outgrow picky eating, but clinicians need to know more so they can, first, *do no harm*, and second, help parents help their children. For now, you need to be aware that many clinicians *don't* know enough, so you can protect yourself and your child from poor advice. Also know that it's okay to find a new doctor or therapist if yours isn't well informed, or is unwilling to learn.

Pressure Tactics and Counterproductive Feeding

Our next stop on the worry cycle is one of the most important: identifying counterproductive feeding tactics, including pressure. These two key questions can help you know if what you are doing constitutes pressure:

1. Why are you doing it? If the answer is to *make* your child eat more (Satter 2014) or try a food (or lick it, or smell it), then it will likely be felt as pressure.

2. How does your child react? If your child shuts down, protests, turns away, whines, negotiates, gets anxious, gags, or vomits, it's probably pressure, no matter how innocuous your action (such as praising him, or asking him to poke a food) might seem.

Forcing or bribing creates pressure, but have you considered that "positive" tactics like praise or sticker charts can create pressure too? Here are examples of pressuring messages or tactics, in seven basic categories.

1. Praise

    "What a big boy, you ate all your _____!"

    "I'm so proud of you for eating _____."

    Sticker charts

    Clapping and cheering

2. Shame or Guilt

    "You asked me to make noodles, now eat it."

    "All the other kids will be eating pizza."

    "If you loved me you would eat this."

    "You ate it before, you'll be fine!"

    "Please be a good girl and take a bite for Mommy!"

3. Bribes

    Child must eat two bites of nonpreferred food before she can have safe or preferred food.

    Child must eat two bites to earn dessert.

Child is paid with cash or toys for eating a specified food or amount.

Child receives a certain amount of video game or TV time per bite.

4. Distraction

    TV, video, or iPad used to get the child to eat.

    Toys used as a distraction (or reward).

    Parents entertain to get child to eat.

5. Threats or Force

    Use of restraint.

    Force-feeding.

    Child is not allowed to leave the table until she eats.

    Holding a spoon in front of the child until she eats.

    "If you don't eat, Daddy will be mad."

6. Pressuring Therapy (including playful in nature)

    Use of spit bowls (child is made to put food in his mouth and then spit it out).

    Child is made to kiss food.

    Child is made to touch or paint with food when he doesn't want to.

7. Nutrition Admonitions

    "You need more _____" (protein, vitamins, and so on).

    "Don't you want to be big and strong?"

    "It's good for you."

Some of the above approaches may not always pose a problem. Take a school program that insists children try one small bite of a new food each day for ten days. This might successfully introduce new foods to an easygoing child who eats well overall (though we believe children can learn to like different foods without such programs). But it might also backfire spectacularly when the child with EPE vomits in front of his classmates.

> **Food for Thought:** Did any of the above tactics work for you? For how long? Did you, for example, have to up the ante for bribes or rewards (more money, bigger toys)?

For Jenny's pickier child, any request to "try one tiny bite" resulted in immediate tears. Though sticker charts helped him complete chores with pride and satisfaction, when his big brother suggested a chart for trying foods, he freaked out. If having spit bowls or a sticker chart has helped your child learn to enjoy a greater variety of foods, we are glad—though if that were the case you probably wouldn't be reading this book.

Our clients' children have tended to react negatively to pressure or encouragement, and studies (including Galloway et al. 2006) demonstrate that this result is common. We know of kids sneaking new foods off the counter or from someone else's bowl when no one is looking, then going into another room (or a closet!) to try it—simply *having someone watch* while they explored the new food was too much pressure. So our list of pressuring tactics, above, is broad.

Many of the above examples of pressure messages or tactics are attempts by adults to get children to comply using logic. Stressed parents may wonder why a seven-year-old who can explain how a computer circuit board works can't or won't understand that he needs calcium for his bones—and eat it. It is tempting to try to explain or convince. But extreme picky eating isn't a problem you can talk or rationalize away—we wish it were so simple.

Sometimes, when talking and bribing fails, parents resort to or are advised to use extreme pressure. If a child is restrained, sobbing, or vomiting due to forced eating, or appears upset or panicked, that is *extreme pressure*, which usually feels upsetting to both the child and the parent engaging in or observing it. We have seen therapy videos of children made to eat "expelled food," which is food that has been partially or wholly swallowed then gagged or vomited up. This is extreme pressure. "Gently guiding" a spoon into a tearful child's mouth by pushing on her jaw when she is clamping her mouth shut is extreme pressure. Professional approaches vary regarding the use of praise, rewards, or reinforcements, but there is a general consensus among feeding professionals that forcing or restraining a child is traumatizing and not helpful.

Sometimes, even what seems like minimal pressure is felt as extreme. Your child's reaction will let you know. Three-year-old Alicia would scream hysterically and often vomit when asked to kiss a banana chip during sessions with her therapist. For Alicia, kissing the banana chip was extreme pressure.

Why Parents Pressure—and Why Kids Push Back

In our experience, these are the main reasons why parents pressure their children to eat:

- They were told to by family, friends, spouses, doctors, or therapists with advice or messages like "Make him eat it" or "Your son can go three weeks without eating and be fine" (this from a pediatrician, no less—a child might *survive* up to three weeks, but how would that feel?) or "She has to eat twenty ounces a day" or "Follow her around with food. Let her eat anything she wants anytime."

- It "works"—at least in the short term, to get one or two bites in.

- They are scared (worried, anxious, terrified—take your pick).

- It's how parents themselves were fed and how much of North America feeds kids.

Parents have a deep-rooted need to nourish. With no obvious alternative, coercion is a natural reaction to a child who resists eating. She needs to eat, after all!

Kids push back against felt pressure for a variety of reasons, including a desire for bodily autonomy or independence, a mismatch between temperament and tactics, and in some cases because conflict is the familiar, safe pattern. Again, let's look at it from the child's point of view.

Bodily Autonomy: "It's my body!"

The most basic reason children resist is because they want to stay comfortable and maintain bodily autonomy and safe boundaries. For example, when a bottle or spoon is forced into an infant's mouth, or his head is held in place while he's attempting to latch or get food in, he may arch his back, turn his head, cry, or bat at the spoon or bottle. Older infants and toddlers may try to get down from or resist the highchair after pressured feedings.

Exercises: Notice how you feel in these scenarios illuminating bodily autonomy.

- *Have someone else brush your teeth. If your child is old enough, ask him to do so. Did you pull back or gag? Were you scared you might get poked?*

- *Have an adult feed you with your eyes closed, presenting an unexpected food with an unexpected utensil (a large wooden spoon or a teaspoon).*

- *Have an adult feed you again (with your eyes open). Try different foods, including one that needs chewing. Have the adult*

*feed you with arbitrary timing, like a bite every three seconds,
even if you are still chewing, or only every thirty seconds.*

- *Finally, work with your feeder to get the timing and utensils the
way you like them.*

A child communicates his need for autonomy through poor
behavior at the table, food refusal, or choosing foods he can safely and
comfortably eat.

Independence: "You can't make me!"

Another reason kids push back is because they are *supposed* to.
Think back to the developmental stages that the toddler, school-aged
child, and tweens and teens go through. Children partly define themselves by opposing their parents. So if parents push the child to eat
broccoli, that's an opportunity to declare independence by saying no.
Depending on the child's history, challenges, and temperament, some
children would rather not eat than lose the battle or face fear or
discomfort.

While your primary concern is likely extreme picky eating, you
may also have a child with a larger than average appetite. The common
approach in getting the child to eat less, by saying something like
"You only need one pork chop," may be met with a rebellious "Oh
yeah? I'm eating three!" When parents pressure children to eat, lick,
or play with a food, take "two more" bites, or eat *less*, the response is
likely to be the opposite of what the parents are trying to achieve.

Over time, the conflict becomes less about food and more about
the battle. As sixteen-year-old Yiseth (with EPE) said, "It shouldn't be
'How can I get her to try this,' but 'How can I help my child do this
at her own pace?'" (Rowell 2012). If children have to "lose" to try a
new food, some will be more interested in the battle. And conflict at
the dinner table can spill into the rest of your relationship with your
child and vice versa. In the words of one heartbroken mother, "It feels
like he hates me."

> **Food for Thought:** How have your child's feeding problems affected your relationship with him? How much daily conflict is about what or how much he eats?

Children who have experienced trauma, or who are building relationships and attachment, may also seek conflict because it feels safe and predictable. If conflict is the default for how your family relates, family counseling can improve this dynamic.

Feelings of Incompetence: "I can't, so why bother trying?"

School-aged children generally want to please and feel capable, but the child with EPE can't and doesn't feel confident when it comes to food. Pressure and attention stall the process, and many children push back, growing increasingly resentful. As clinician and author Madeline Levine explained in a 2012 *New York Times* article, "Continued, unnecessary intervention makes your child feel bad about himself (if he's young) or angry at you (if he's a teenager)." If they can't meet expectations, why bother trying?

Temperament Matters

Coexisting with developmentally appropriate desires for autonomy, independence, and competence, temperament is an often overlooked factor determining a child's reaction to feeding tactics—there is no one-size-fits-all solution. An easygoing child might accept a "no-thank-you" bite with "You were right—I like parsnips!" while the same rule results in a tantrum or sulking for an independent, strong-willed, anxious, or cautious child. Your child's reactions will guide your feeding decisions.

The Pressure Paradox: Even If You Win, Everyone Loses

With all the effort, negotiating, and bribes, why aren't things better? It may seem that the more you struggle, the worse feeding goes, like being stuck in quicksand. When children learn to eat for the wrong reasons, there can be serious, unintended consequences. Pressure may give you the short-term victory of getting in one or two bites or feeling in control, but it will come at the cost of your child eating (or not) for reasons other than hunger, fullness, or appetite. This is the paradox of pressure. You may win the battle but lose the war.

Kids Learn to Eat for the Wrong Reasons

If children eat to please you, to avoid punishment, or to earn a toy, that reinforces *external* motivation, and they learn to eat for the wrong reasons. Over time, when children (or adults) eat without regard to internal cues like hunger or appetite, they can lose touch with those cues. We can feed children in ways that support and nurture inborn skills of self-regulation, or we can feed them in ways that bury those skills. (We say "bury" and not "eliminate" skills, as we have seen children learn to tune in even after very difficult beginnings.)

Pressure Increases Anxiety and Decreases Appetite

Anxiety, fear, and conflict turn off appetite and make children eat and grow less well. Many resources acknowledge that anxiety turns off appetite, but so can less subtle pressure, like watchful eyes on a reluctant eater or expecting an older child to keep a tasting journal.

When you preplate food, your child may become upset and anxious about the food in front of him and preoccupied with negotiating: how many bites must he take? How long can he watch TV or play video games? Stress hormones surge, and appetite—or any budding curiosity about food—disappears. At such times, children literally can't sense hunger or fullness signals from their bodies because too much else is going on. Stress and panic activate the fight-or-flight response, decreasing saliva production (making food harder to swallow and changing taste perception), and digestion slows significantly in the stomach and gut, interfering with and confusing appetite and hunger signals.

Many moms challenge the idea that stress and anxiety decrease appetite, citing that they themselves eat more when stressed. For many adults who have dieted or experienced food insecurity, negative emotions generally do lead to *eating more*; this is also the case for children who have had their intake restricted. The vast majority of children with EPE have not been restricted, and we agree with the consensus that negative emotions decrease their appetite and intake.

It's notable that some children *can* be taught to *overeat* when encouraged. One example is premature babies, who start life very small and whose caregivers expend a lot of effort getting them to eat more. These children may end up at a higher weight in adolescence than full-term babies (Vasylyeva et al. 2013). More research is needed, but the findings so far are consistent with our observations and those of our colleagues working with NICU grads. It appears that some children resist pressure and eat less, while others follow encouragement and learn to eat more than they otherwise would. We don't yet understand why (temperament probably plays a role), but we believe that trying to get children to eat more than they want leads children to lose touch with internal cues and promotes problems with weight regulation at both extremes.

Pressure Makes Kids Like Food Less

Parents may think they're helping by bribing with dessert, but research suggests this can backfire in two important ways: 1) children learn to value and desire the dessert even more; and 2) they learn to like the other foods less (Newman and Taylor 1992).

Consider this scene at a buffet. Three adults are focused on making a young boy eat two bites of chicken to earn dessert. The adults sit grim-faced, chiming in about how good the chicken is, only two bites, he can plug his nose, he needs more protein, it's good for him… No one talks about anything else. The boy whines and stalls.

After about twenty minutes, he has one bite, which is deemed good enough, and an adult fetches dessert. Everyone smiles, oohing and aahing over the donuts, generally having a grand time: they have gone from misery to rainbows and puppies. This boy has learned that chicken is endured to get to the *good* stuff!

The aversive effects of pressure can be long term. One study showed that college students overwhelmingly disliked foods they were forced to eat as children (Batsell et al. 2002). One parent, describing herself as a picky child, now eats almost everything but still hates milk—because her parents consistently pushed it. When parents oversell, pressure, push, and bribe children to eat certain foods, children may think, "This must not be very good if my parents are working so hard to get me to eat it."

Pressure Makes Kids Depend on You (or a Device) for Every Bite

Some parents find themselves with children who *only* eat with distractions like screens or toys, or with the threat of withholding toys or affection. In fact, many behavioral therapies teach this approach and even keep children from feeding themselves, insisting that parents control every aspect of every bite. While parents may have short-term success getting calories in with this approach, families often wind up with a child heading to preschool or kindergarten unable unable to eat without the parent (or iPad) present.

Jenny worked with a mom whose daughter (with no identified special needs) attended an inpatient feeding program followed by outpatient therapy where Mom had to feed every bite from a spoon. A year later, the daughter ate only yogurt and blended ravioli from Mom's spoon while distracted with a movie, and Mom had no idea how to transition to age-appropriate eating. Many children need support as they develop eating skills and may take longer to reach goals, but trying to fast-track the process by relying on tactics that create dependence works against typical development. When social and emotional health and development are sacrificed to achieve nutrition and weight goals, it erodes trust and the child's sense of competence, and backfires more often than not.

The Lure of Behavioral Modification

Many of you have already tried rewards, toys, bribes, sticker charts, videos used as reinforcement, "take a bite" rules, or punishment. Jenny's extensive experience with behavioral feeding approaches and familiarity with the research led her to conclude that behavioral modification often works best for more concrete tasks. A toy or sticker as reward may help a child get through homework, potty train, or make his bed. Speech and feeding, however, are complex tasks, and the reward approach is less suited for say, the development of natural-sounding, functional language or of long-term enjoyment of eating. We've both heard as much from parents: "Video game bribes work for everything but eating." No amount of external rewards can bring your child with EPE to the point of eating and enjoying something if she is not ready.

> **Food for Thought:** Someone offers you $10,000 to eat eight ounces of your own vomit. You really want the money, but could you do it?

When an approach works well for some tasks, it is tempting to try to make it work for eating. If you're recognizing that rewards and bribes aren't helping, honor your observations. Your child's reaction is the best evidence of whether a strategy is successful.

In this chapter, we've taken you on one round of the worry cycle. You've probably noticed that the cycle intensifies: more worry leads to increased pressure, your child resists more forcefully with every turn, and you're stuck. It's time to get unstuck—starting with the sense of relief that comes from knowing you don't have to *get* your child to eat. With your foundation of understanding of what is typical and how and where children and parents can get off track, you are empowered to stop the cycle and support your child's eating and growth. The rest of this book will show you how.

CHAPTER 4

Step 1: Decrease Anxiety, Stress, and Power Struggles

Now that you've gained a foundation for thinking about feeding, it's time to tackle step 1: reducing anxiety, stress, and power struggles. Even if you manage to get everyone sitting down to a "perfect" home-cooked meal, progress will be minimal until you take anxiety off the table. In this chapter, we suggest ways to reduce anxiety (yours and your child's), which is the key to helping your child feel good about eating, and to helping him eat the right amount and variety for good health.

Understanding and Addressing Your Anxiety

Patterns of thoughts, emotions, and behaviors, over time, create neural pathways in the brain. Think of wagon wheels on a dirt road back in pioneer days: as the road was traveled countless times, deep grooves, or ruts, formed in the dirt. Wagons traveled easily in the grooves, but great effort was required to forge a new path—and if just one wheel ran into a rut, the whole wagon fell back in the old grooves. If a child has experienced anxiety around food, maybe gagging while trying to eat those two bites for months or years, that negative association is reinforced and gagging becomes the automatic response to mealtimes—the child is stuck in a rut. And if you've ever learned to do something the "wrong" way, like swim, swing a golf club, or type, you know that unlearning that pattern is much harder than learning how to do it the "right" way from the start because you are fighting established neural pathways and muscle memory.

The wagon wheel analogy helps explain the frustrating scenario wherein a child gags or panics out of the blue, as if a switch has been flipped. Take for example the child who may be chatting about soccer while eating something she hasn't tried for months. Four bites in, a look of fear descends, the color drains from her face, and she may even gag. The parents think, "We know you can do this—you just did!" What they might not realize is that something (encouragement, a full bowl, a feeling on the back of the tongue) triggered the child's anxious response—those wagon wheels really want to get back into the familiar grooves!

Bruce Perry of the Child Trauma Academy explains that even minor triggers can lead to "full-blown response patterns (e.g. hyper-arousal or dissociation)" (Perry et al. 1995, 275). It takes time for new experiences to lay down new neural pathways. The good news is that children's brains are quite plastic, or changeable, and more easily form new tracks than adult brains do.

Exercise: Visualize the above scenario (the girl gagging four bites in) and practice a neutral reaction (one mom called it her "pleasant poker face"). If your child gags or vomits, stay calm and take a breath. Try your best not to express distress or frustration in front of your child.

What Is Making You Anxious?

On a scale of one to ten, parents commonly describe their anxiety and stress around feeding as eleven. You have your own neural pathways around feeding—a sense of dread before meals, or falling into the same automatic response. You are likely stuck in a rut too. Your child takes cues from you, so reducing *your* anxiety will help hers, and will start you down the road to new neural pathways.

In the last chapter we reviewed some common worries about nutrition, and next we'll explore other sources of stress and anxiety. A 2013 article by Clarissa Martin and colleagues, "Maternal Stress and Problem-Solving," explains how mothers of children with picky eating report more mealtime stress, which leads to less creative problem solving and increased pressure, which can increase food refusal (there's that worry cycle again!).

Food for Thought: Identifying your own fears and feelings about picky eating is the place to start addressing anxiety. You may even have called picky eaters "annoying" in the past, vowing you would never raise one! What emotions do the following issues bring up?

Judgment from others (parents, friends, family, medical professionals)

Your child's growth or nutrition

Your child being teased or ostracized for how he eats

Your child's discomfort or anxiety around food

Nutrition concerns

Are there issues not on the list that you feel fear and anxiety about? Ask your partner to identify his or her own fears so you are aware of and can empathize with each other's concerns. If you and your partner aren't on the same page with feeding, that is its own source of stress.

When Parents Disagree

When parents disagree or argue over feeding, each loses the benefit of a supportive partner, and they may see increased conflict at meals, making an already difficult job harder. Also, when parents have different rules, the mixed messages fuel anxiety for the child unsure of whose rules apply when. The parent who walks in the door at six to sit down to dinner often doesn't understand the frustration, effort, and anxiety involved in getting meals and snacks together (along with everything else) day after day. Finally, children know when parents aren't united and may try to use that to their advantage. (Think about a teen asking the more lenient parent for permission to go to a concert: "Dad said yes!")

Please excuse our generalized observations, but we find that fathers often want to "fix" the problem and make eating happen, tending to cling to pressuring rules. At the same time, though, we note that fathers seem less bothered by feeding problems and are more relaxed overall. Parenting differences can be positive for children as long as they don't generate a great deal of tension, and especially if parents can appreciate each other's strengths. Examining your parenting styles and leaning on your partner can benefit your relationship and your children. It may be hard to admit, but your partner may have a healthier approach. For example, if one parent has an eating disorder, it may be better for now for the child to eat with the parent who has a healthier relationship to food.

Food for Thought: Talk to your partner about what meals were like when you each were little. Do you think how you were raised around food helped you have a healthy relationship with food? Were you forced to eat? Think about how your *experiences as children* have shaped how you approach mealtimes today.

If parents aren't approaching feeding the same way, many have still found success when one parent "drives the bus" while the other is supportive (even if only by agreeing to keep silent). Seeing progress is what often helps both parents get on board.

Seek Common Ground and Understanding

If possible, read this book with your partner or share the exercises and Food for Thought sections. Keep an open dialogue. Sharing how Maddy didn't cry before breakfast, or that she drank from a mug or dipped her bread in lentil soup, can help others recognize progress and the primary caregiver to feel supported. Celebrate successes together—just not in front of the kids!

Sometimes uncovering a resistant parent's motivation helps. One dad explained that he thinks it shows respect for his wife if everyone eats what she prepares. When his wife shared that her priority was enjoying their time at the table, rather than negotiating bites, it helped Dad ease up on the rules he grew up with. Instead, Dad and the kids thanked Mom for cooking (and they cleaned up!). (It's nice to thank the cook, whether it's Mom, Dad, the kids, or the cook at the local diner!)

If your partner doesn't trust the process yet, letting go of old rules will be tough, especially if doctors and others still push or if your partner hasn't had his or her worries addressed. Reflecting on everything you've tried that hasn't worked can help. Journaling is a great way to do this. (Have you started yet?)

Two or More Households

If two or even three households (say, divorced parents and a grandparent providing child care) are involved, conflicts can multiply. When arrangements are complex, it can be beneficial to find a family therapist whom all involved parties can trust. Focusing on the well-being of the child, and responding to her cues, will help caregivers determine the best approach. Maintaining as stable a routine as possible between and among the households also reduces anxiety all around.

Judgment

Being judged by others, especially friends, family, or your child's teachers, can feel like getting kicked when you're down. Judgment from medical and therapy professionals can feel the worst, because you want to be seen as a good client and a good parent. One couple Jenny worked with had devoted endless hours to help their son eat more, with over three hundred mealtime DVDs and a room full of reward toys. All that effort resulted in a little boy fed by a tube and refusing all food by mouth. The parents had been told by the previous feeding team that they had failed *because they were holding the spoon too high when they put it to his mouth.* More likely this approach failed because the scared father, feeling it was his fault, became more determined to get the minimum amount in and resorted to force-feeding—with his son then vomiting multiple times per day.

You *will* be judged. Sometimes people will want to help by offering suggestions, books, or tips, but it still feels like judgment. Remind yourself as often as possible that every parent struggles, even the one judging you right now. Here are some ways to find some relief from the judging:

- Seek support from other parents who are going through what you are. There are private Facebook groups that are moderated to protect participants.

- Avoid Internet or media stories that make you feel bad: take a social media break, quit discussion boards.

- When close friends or family offer what they think is helpful advice, ask them instead to listen. Parents often share with us how important it is to have someone just listen and not judge or offer help.

Here is some language you can use or adapt to ask for what you need. Say: **"I know you want to help, but I really need someone to listen."** Or **"We really have tried everything. Please don't send** links to articles or recipes anymore." Or **"I'm so glad you want to help. Could you take Cori to her piano lesson so I can run a few errands?"**

The Stress of Feeding Therapy

Juggling therapy appointments can make an already hectic life feel out of control. Research shows that parents in behavioral feeding therapy often employ multiple strategies to get a child to eat, like TV, toys, or other rewards, and enforcing numbers of bites. Talk about balls in the air! Parents with children in inpatient behavioral therapy also exhibit increased stress, likely due to the strict and time-consuming protocols (Didehbani et al. 2011).

Parents admit that they they often stop going to therapy because the assigned tasks didn't feel right, were too hard, or took too long. Rather than realizing the therapy itself wasn't a fit, parents often feel (and may be told) that they aren't working hard enough, especially if children succeed with skills during therapy sessions but feeding at home is still a struggle—a sign that you need more or different support (which we explore in chapter 8).

On the other hand, some parents have said, "Just tell us what to do!" A task-by-task protocol or two-bite rule may give you a sense of control, which can reduce stress—and may even work initially. It's important to acknowledge how tempting that sense of relief can be. Sometimes the less linear STEPS+ approach can take some getting used to, with fewer spelled-out tasks and an emphasis on relearning and supporting normal eating, however long it takes. With time, you will develop a *feeling of competence* as you learn to make decisions and be your child's best support. That feeling of competence will help you trust yourself, your child, and the process.

Anxiety Around Meltdowns or Tantrums

One mom shared that a paralyzing fear of her son's intense and lengthy tantrums dictated how she fed. This fear may be particularly potent if your child has tantrums to the point of vomiting. But hoping to make changes without any resistance isn't realistic. If your child knows you will give in to any demand to avoid a tantrum, he has control. Seek help from books, family therapists, or local parent educators in dealing with tantrums if they are holding you hostage. Realize that STEPS+ tends to *help* with behavior, though you can't avoid all tantrums.

Anxiety Around Lack of Control

Many of us find it profoundly unsettling when we don't feel in control. If your child has that same yearning for control, it may make for epic battles. Sometimes the only end to the struggle is to let go of the rope you are both tugging on. This doesn't mean walking away; it means accepting how little real control you have over how much he eats. Scary stuff, but ending the struggle helps him eat better in the long run. An unknown author said, "We cannot direct the wind but we can adjust the sails"—in other words, your anxiety may never fully go away, but how you respond *is* in your control. Working to understand and lessen your anxiety—along with establishing a routine, having family meals, and building skills—is within your control.

Lessening Your Anxiety

Anxiety is fueled when we feel out of control, fear losing control, or struggle to gain control of the uncontrollable. The opposite of the need for control is faith. "Faith is taking the first step even when you don't see the whole staircase," as Martin Luther King Jr. is believed to have said. Right now you might feel unable to visualize what's at the end of STEPS+: a family meal that you and your kids look forward to, with everyone eating and enjoying food together. Put your worry and anxiety on the back burner for now, and cultivate the faith that you'll sit down to that meal one day.

It can be useful to think of helping your child learn to eat as like tending tulips. There is much you can do: prep the soil, mulch and fertilize, and plant the bulb in a sunny spot. Then you hope for the best. When the shoot comes up in the spring, you weed and water; and if you try to pry open the bud before it's ready, you may damage or destroy the flower. Like the tulip, your child's eating will flourish in time—with the proper environment, and with your support.

But how can you cultivate your faith when anxiety and stress are so much more familiar?

Accepting Where You Are Right Now

Start by unconditionally accepting what and how much your child eats. As blogger Skye Van Zetten (2013) wrote, "Step back and meet your child's eating needs where they are right now. If crackers are the only acceptable food she finds on the table, let her eat as many crackers as she wants with your blessings. Learning to trust your child with eating is a process that involves letting go of everything you've been taught and told about feeding your family."

Try these tips to reduce your anxiety and cultivate acceptance:

- Stop counting calories (delete that phone app) and doing daily weigh-ins. If you wouldn't do anything differently based on the information you are gathering, *stop*.

- If you are weighing your child, particularly if your child is older, make it quick and matter-of-fact, maybe right before or after a bath. Consider only weighing once a week.

- Question consultants who push daily calorie minimums, or find new ones who will support you in thinking about intake over several days or a week.

- Find your own version of the sentiments in the famous Serenity Prayer: *Let me accept the things I cannot control* (challenges, how much of what foods he eats, how long it will take), *the courage to change the things I can* (routines, what I say and do, family meals), *and the wisdom to know the difference.*

- When your anxiety peaks, take action to bring it down. Take deep breaths, take an herbal tea break, hold your partner's hand at the table, skip or cut back on caffeine, go for a walk, see a therapist, learn relaxation techniques, put on your favorite music and dance: whatever works for you.

- If you're overwhelmed at the table, calmly excuse yourself for a few moments (provided your child is safe to be left alone or your partner is there). Come back when you're ready.

- Go to your child's favorite restaurant and let him order what he wants, even if it's only fries. Make having a nice time the goal, and savor that feeling.

- Let go of your timetable. If you want your child eating "normally" in six weeks, you'll fail.

But accepting your child and managing your anxieties will be impossible if you fear that your child is or will be unhealthy. While we've addressed basic nutrition fears, your biggest fear may be that your child will lose weight or need a feeding tube, and might even die—and it's time to address this fear head on.

Facing the Fear That Your Child Will Lose Weight

The main obstacle for many parents is the worry that their child will lose weight. Unaddressed, this fear undermines your trust in the STEPS+ process and in your child. The fear of weight loss drives the extreme efforts to get those two bites in, and it may feel scary to stop pressuring. It is hard for parents to accept that overall, pressure *decreases* intake. Your child might indeed eat less for a few days or weeks, which is why we recommend you read the whole book before jumping in. If you don't fully understand the process or know how to handle challenges, your fear will push you into your familiar neural pathways (your rut) and you'll be back in that worry cycle.

In our experience with the transition away from pressuring tactics, when we see intake go down, it is usually for a few days or weeks before anxiety decreases, appetite kicks in, cues are learned, and intake rises. As long as the steps are in place, with at least one safe food at every meal and snack, what we see *most* often is a rather quick increase in intake, of at least the safe foods. Many children begin to experience an increase in appetite, and weight stabilizes or even increases within a few weeks.

Consider three-year-old Amari, who had gained nine ounces the previous year. Her mom was skeptical, but within three days of her removing pressure and putting other steps into place, the daily vomiting and gagging Amari had experienced for several weeks stopped. Ten days in, Mom noted one larger meal a day and Amari's anxiety improved. Though Mom was still scared about Amari's weight, she hung in there, and a few weeks later the pocketing (food kept between the cheeks and gums) disappeared. Six weeks later, Amari had gained more weight than in the previous year, and within six months she was on the growth charts for the first time.

Not all children fit this scenario. One parent, whose son had lengthy and severe food anxieties starting in infancy, reported that while his child became much happier, calmer, and more interested in food, he continued to have comparatively low intake for two years. In this case, however, the important thing was that the child was growing, thriving in all other areas, and learning how to eat for his own body's needs.

For children who are medically fragile, have extreme anxiety or complex feeding histories, or are weaning off feeding tubes, you might see weight loss, and a more cautious or gradual approach may help. This might include using supplements or calorie additives for a time, including more safe foods at meals than you would otherwise, and staying in close contact with your child's health care team. We always recommend that your child be followed by health and nutrition professionals who can assess reductions in intake and how your child is doing overall.

Rarely, a child will not eat enough by mouth even when pressure is removed. In our experience, this usually indicates other factors at play, such as unknown or inadequately addressed medical issues or anxiety, significant strain in the parent-child relationship, or poor reserves of strength and nutrition to tolerate even a slight decrease in intake. Sometimes a feeding tube is the best solution, as it removes the pressure around oral intake while supporting nutrition. As one mom wrote in an email, "I've imagined rock bottom, and that's a feeding tube, but it can't be worse than this." (Feeding tubes also support children who aspirate food into the lungs or who have a metabolic disease where even trace amounts of certain foods, or an improper balance, could lead to brain damage or death.)

Some clinicians improperly use tubes from the nose to the stomach (nasogastric or NG tubes). Taped to the cheeks, these tubes are uncomfortable, often worsening aversions, and should only be used for specific, short-term (one to two weeks) situations. A tube directly to the stomach through the abdominal wall, known as a gastrostomy tube, G-tube, or button, is preferred if poor intake is chronic. You may have the impression that a feeding tube is drastic and to be avoided at all costs. Unfortunately, clinicians have been known to threaten parents with a tube, exaggerating the negatives, in a mis-guided attempt to motivate parents to get the child to eat.

But a feeding tube is not a failure; rather, it gives a child time to learn to eat at her own pace while meeting nutritional needs, and provides relief to parents worried about intake. One dad shared, "Learning that there's a stomach feeding tube option, which isn't *that* terrible, took a lot of stress off." Not a single parent we worked with who decided on a feeding tube regretted the decision. When children are ready, the tube is removed. For a very few, it may be needed for some years. As Suzanne Evans Morris explained in a personal communication, "Incorporating feeding tubes into meal routines as simply an alternative or additional way to feed a child helps children and families develop a positive relationship with food and mealtimes and a delight in whatever they are able to eat orally." For more on feeding tubes, see the "Resources" page at the website associated with this book, http://www.newharbinger.com/31106.

Understanding and Lessening Your Child's Anxiety

Your child with EPE may feel anxious, defeated, and incapable, leaving you walking on eggshells to keep the peace. In a 2012 study, Farrow and Coulthard noted that "the characteristics of sensory sensitivity (e.g., noticing small perceptual changes, a tendency to respond negatively to change) may be markers of higher child anxiety which then predict greater negativity in the context of food" (845). Sensory sensitivity, anxiety, and "greater negativity" around food appear to go hand in hand. Many children are unable to express feelings with words, so here are some signs that your child may be anxious around food:

- Whining or crying

- Gagging at the sight of food

- Refusing to come to the table

- Avoidant body positioning (leaning back, turning away)

- Dissociating or tuning out: looks "glazed" or "zoned out"

- Flushed or pale skin

- Shaking, tapping, or rocking

- Talking too much or not at all

- Consistently poor behavior at the table

This list helps you identify what situations cause your child anxiety. Watch your child for any of these (or other) signs to start to understand his triggers.

Reassure Her That She Doesn't Have to Eat

The best way to reduce your child's anxiety is to address your own so that you can stop pressuring. But that might not be enough. One client shared that her daughter seemed interested in new foods, but kept asking, "Will you make me try it?" A year and a half earlier, a feeding therapist had repeatedly restrained and fed the girl while she screamed. Mom was instructed to do the same at home, which was so upsetting that they stopped after a few tries. Eighteen months later, this little girl still didn't trust that she wouldn't be forced. Help your child overcome this anxiety by acknowledging past pressure. Get down on her level, ask questions, listen, and promise she won't be forced again—if you mean it. Here is some language that may help you understand your child's anxiety and reassure her that you won't make her eat: **"Why do you say that?" "Are you afraid I'll make you try it?" "Can you tell me what you mean?"** Or say: **"In this family, no one has to eat (touch/play with/lick) anything they don't want to."** Or **"We used to ask you to touch food and put it on your plate. We won't ask you to do that anymore."**

Even if you didn't restrain your child, if you enforced bite rules or made her sit until she finished, she doesn't trust yet that you won't make her eat. Telling her in clear terms that you won't make her eat, lick, or kiss any food is step one, but what really helps is when you follow through and consistently let her decide how much and what to eat, even if it's only crackers for a while.

Let Him Know There Will Always Be Something He Can Eat

Does your child ask repeatedly what's for dinner? Is he preoccupied with the menu on the way to a friend's birthday party? The need to know what will be served is natural for a child with EPE: he's seeking reassurance that he will be able to eat something.

In the past your child might have arrived hungry at a playdate or party, with no safe foods to eat. Friends' parents may have even pressured him to eat, making him more anxious about not eating or not fitting in. Every time Jenny goes to a social gathering with her younger son, he asks if and what they will be eating. Children may even ask to skip family gatherings and social functions to avoid this stress. Understand and try to ease this anxiety in your child. These phrases may help:

"We will find something you can eat."

"I believe that you'll find something you can eat. I called ahead, and they are having cake and ice cream and pizza."

"We'll bring chips and salsa to the party. You can enjoy the chips and see what else they have."

"We'll eat at home after the party, so it's okay if there's nothing you want to eat here."

"Susie's mom is serving pretzels."

In chapter 7 we go into planning what foods to serve and finding success away from home, but for now, know that reassuring your child that he won't go hungry helps his anxiety. You can also allow him to eat before you go out if you don't know what is being served. Enjoying the social scene is the goal for now—though sometimes your child may surprise you and try new things away from home!

Reassure Her You Won't Be Disappointed If She Doesn't Eat

Your child may feel she is disappointing you at every meal, which can lead to high levels of anxiety. To her, she is failing at something you both want her to be good at. (A child less concerned with pleasing you may not have this heightened sense of failure.) The old adage "Success breeds success" works the other way too—failure can breed failure. When your child sees disappointment on your face at every eating opportunity, she may feel like *nothing* she does is enough and stop trying. Eating new things takes courage; you want to bolster that courage and limit her feelings of failure. When you accept her how she is now, letting go of expectations for her eating, and focus on enjoying her company, she will pick up on that.

It may seem counterintuitive, but try *not praising* your child's eating even if she makes progress. Praising her today communicates that if she doesn't feel brave tomorrow, she has disappointed you. Praise can be another form of pressure. Children do best relying on *internal motivation* to eat, rather than eating for approval. Kids who are used to praise often ask for it initially. You can still be positive and responsive with **"Oh, you tried the carrots? I'm happy you're happy!"** or **"I enjoy them too! We can make them this way again soon."**

Here are a few ideas to help your child know that you believe in her and know that she is capable.

Do:

- Give mealtime jobs: wash veggies, shake salt into pasta water, stir foods, set a timer, lay the table, and so on; older kids can light a candle.

- Enjoy his company. Try to ignore what and how much he eats.

- Keep exposing her to new flavors and foods. Katja overheard a dad with his young daughter at the grocery store say, "But you don't like strawberries, you don't like blueberries…" He reinforced what she "didn't like," and not buying the berries denied her the opportunity to get used to different foods.

Don't:

- Label your child as "the picky eater."

- Lower expectations. "You won't like anything here, but you can fill up on bread." Even if he only eats bread, don't set him up to fail. Tonight may be the night he decides to try something.

- Talk about his eating in front of him. Discreetly keep an eye on intake or talk privately with your spouse, doctor, or nanny. Children are great at listening when we don't think they are (and not so great at it when we ask them to clean their rooms).

- Look in her lunchbox or ask what she ate for lunch *first thing* when you pick her up. Send the message that what she ate is not the most important thing.

- Allow criticism of others' food choices or foods on the table. **"Don't yuck my yum"** is a great phrase we've heard. This goes for the whole family. Mom can't say "gross" to Dad's choices either.

Your child doesn't trust herself with eating yet either, so lead by example: tell her and show her that you believe she can and will learn to eat more of a variety of foods when she is ready.

If Your Child Needs Help with Anxiety

If you are concerned your child may need help with anxiety, addressing anxiety *separate from food issues* may be best; there is research that supports this approach. Relaxation exercises or biofeedback aimed at reducing anxiety while looking at or touching a spider may help with a spider phobia, but we find that using this approach to deal with food fears often backfires. This "exposure" or "flooding" therapy with nonpreferred or challenging foods often makes extreme picky eating worse: these are the kids vomiting or crying in the parking lot outside the therapy building.

Instead, find a therapist specializing in childhood anxiety, and ask for help with anxiety management or specific anxiety-reduction techniques like mindfulness, not eating. Play therapies may be particularly helpful. (As we discussed earlier, EPE is associated with generalized anxiety and obsessive-compulsive traits.)

Decreasing Power Struggles

A mealtime environment that feels like a battleground hinders your child's progress and undermines your relationship with him. Understanding why certain feeding techniques invite power struggles will help you avoid them. Approaches invite conflict when they:

- Rely on external pressure, such as rewards like videos or toys, or threats of punishment or of being ignored

- Don't help children learn to eat in ways consistent with typical development

- Don't help children learn to feel good around food

- Bury the child's internal regulation signals, making it more likely that she will eat more or less than she needs

Moving away from external motivation (pressure, rewards, praise, rules) and leading your child toward internal motivation (which, keep in mind, is inborn) seems daunting if you have been taught that only *you* can make him eat. We know many families who have gone through feeding therapy programs with short-term success in increasing amounts of purees or calories. But ultimately, the child burns out on the rewards or bribes (if they even worked in the first place), parents tire of the process, and the situation deteriorates.

Accessing internal motivation—the magical "I do it"—neutralizes power struggles. When your child is internally motivated, it's not you making her eat, it's her wanting to. And children really do want to, even if the desire is currently somewhere deep inside. Allowing children to control *whether* and *how much* they eat means they can relax and tap into their internal drive to learn about, taste, and eventually eat more foods.

Know Your Role and Stick to It

The key to supporting your child's internal motivation—neutralizing power struggles and reducing anxiety—is to clearly define your role and your child's. Feeding expert, author, dietitian, and family therapist Ellyn Satter (1986) pioneered the concept of the division of responsibility (DOR) in feeding, the cornerstone you can return to to clarify your respective roles. Increasingly, this nearly thirty-year-old guiding principle of feeding is being backed up by research on feeding styles, "responsive feeding" in particular. In 2011, the *Journal of Nutrition Education and Behavior* even compiled a special edition on "responsive feeding." Here is the DOR in a nutshell:

Your job: decide when, where, and what foods are offered (as long as you include something your child can eat)

Your child's job: decide whether and how much to eat

It sounds simple, but it's not easy, especially early on. When you feel sucked into power struggles, step back and ask yourself: "What's my job? Am I allowing my child to do *my* job? Am I doing *his*?" Consider the preschool pick-up when Katja's then three-year-old had a meltdown over her snack: pears, multigrain crackers, and whipped cream cheese. This public display of her little girl sobbing for a ham sandwich had Katja thinking, "What's the harm? I can make a ham sandwich. That's pretty balanced." Katja reflected on why it felt wrong and realized that 1) the snack included foods her daughter usually enjoyed, 2) her daughter was trying to do Katja's job of deciding what was served, and 3) they were in a power struggle. "Pears and crackers are for snack." Katja said. "I'm sorry you're disappointed; we'll have a ham sandwich soon." The tantrum continued for a few minutes, but they were soon at the park enjoying the planned snack and ready to play.

Exercise: See if you can identify where roles are getting mixed up. (Assume at least one safe food is offered.)

1. *Tim gets up during dinner to get crackers.*

2. *Sophia cries for a pink smoothie, though Mom already added blueberries. Mom tosses the purple smoothie, starting over. Sophia*

demands to have it in front of the TV, but then refuses and asks for French toast.

3. *Dad insists Kevin can't have dessert until he eats at least one bite of everything on his plate.*

Answers: 1. Tim is doing the adult's job of deciding *what* is offered. 2. Mom is allowing Sophia to do Mom's jobs of deciding *what* is served and *where*. 3. Dad is doing Kevin's job of deciding *whether* and *how much* to eat from what is offered, and is pressuring.

Unfortunately, the principles of the DOR have often been misinterpreted and misapplied—even by professionals. Rest assured that it is not "They eat green beans and rice or nothing." When you provide enough of at least one safe food, your child will be able to choose from what is available.

Negotiation blurs the lines of the DOR. If your child thinks that saying the right thing or whining might get her what she wants—but maybe not—that uncertainty increases anxiety. Refusing to negotiate isn't cruel; it reduces anxiety. Try **"I love you too much to argue"** (Fay and Fay 2000).

Prepare Your Child for the New Roles

With a young or preverbal child, make necessary changes and explain only what you need to. If your child is older, tell her how and why things are different. This helps her feel respected and secure, and lets her know what to expect. As you talk to her, focus on connecting with her—on becoming partners as you discuss what isn't working now. You can ask her what she doesn't like about meals. You can acknowledge that what you've tried hasn't helped, and, if it feels authentic to do so, you can apologize. Here are some language suggestions:

"We're a problem-solving family. We'll figure this out together."

"I think we're all tired of the fighting. We're going to do things differently. It might take some getting used to, but we want to have a better time at the table."

"You'll like not having to do spit bowls anymore, but you might not like when we ask you not to get applesauce pouches between meals. That's okay. We learned that eating meals and then waiting for a bit before snacks helps our bodies."

Letting your child know you are in the lead and will take care of her reassures her. Admitting that you are not perfect, and may not get it all right immediately, is okay too.

Protecting Your Child from Pressure from Others

Pressure from others can be a significant source of stress for your child. The feeding approach we describe is not what most Americans are used to. It's helpful to have strategies ready to protect your child from comments from friends and family, teachers, childcare providers, and others. Grandparents, who may have been raised in a time when food was scarce, often seem particularly upset when children won't eat, and may take it personally if their own children seem to reject how they were raised.

Skye Van Zetten of *Mealtime Hostage* once shared on social media how she coped at a community picnic: "I fended off several comments directed at my kids from around the table, 'Aren't you going to eat that/finish that/try that?' My response was to always address my child and ask, 'Are you full?' 'Yes,' they replied. I'm pleased to say that was all it took to make the requests stop."

In the past, you may have asked a sitter or teacher to enforce feeding rules. Explaining a change might feel awkward. You could say something like **"I know we asked you to have Sammy eat her main meal before she could have her dessert, and we appreciate your**

efforts, but we're learning that it's probably making things worse."

If other people frequently eat with your child, have a private discussion with them about your approach (or give them the one-page "Essentials: Helping a Child with Extreme Picky Eating" in the online Resources). Prepare them with the phrase, **"Follow my lead."** Acknowledge that it's not how they might do things, but that it's important they not pressure your child to eat. If they forget and push a "no-thank-you bite," you can intervene, saying something like: **"That's not how we do things. Manny doesn't have to eat anything he doesn't want to."** Or **"He doesn't have to finish his plate. His body knows when he is done eating."** Or **"We don't do 'no-thank-you' bites."** Hopefully this will suffice. Or, as Skye Van Zetten did, simply ask your child, **"Are you full?"** and let his answer deflect pressure.

The language in the scripts above can be adapted to strangers or waitstaff. If others suggest your child shouldn't have dessert until he's finished his meal, try **"We're doing fine here. Please bring his dessert now."** When your child hears you defend him in front of others, it sends a powerful message of trust and gives him words to use to stand up for himself. It amazed a client the first time her daughter confidently refused food pushed on her by a friend's mother, saying, "No thank you, my mom says I don't have to eat anything I don't want to."

Protecting Your Child at School or with Child Care or Nannies

One of Jenny's clients shared that his child's school followed the popular policy that kids must finish the "main food" at lunch first, losing recess if they don't. This greatly increased his son's anxiety, and he ate less and less. (We've heard of kids asking parents not to pack more than a few bites because of rules like these!) In spite of the dad speaking with the principal and a note from the feeding team asking staff not to pressure, the school refused to make any exceptions. In this case, there was little choice but to change schools.

One mom noted that her preschooler came home in spare clothes almost daily due to vomiting. Mom asked the teacher not to make her finish her lunch, and the little girl began coming home in the same clothes she went to school in; things were improving. If you suspect there is a problem away from home and your child can't or won't explain, ask to observe or videotape a meal.

Conversely, children frequently eat better at child care or with nannies. While this may hurt parents' feelings, it is encouraging, because it means a sensory, oral motor, or other physiological problem is less likely. Children save their best and worst for their parents, and sometimes others who aren't as worried or invested may intuitively avoid power struggles.

It's hard to ask children to stand up for themselves with adults. Sometimes a lunchbox card, such as the following, can help. (A printable version of the card is available online at http://www.newharbin ger.com/31106.)

Dear _____ ,

Please don't ask _____ to eat more or different foods than she wants. Please let her eat as much as she wants of any of the foods I pack, in any order, even if she eats nothing, or only dessert. If you have any concerns or questions, please call me at _____ .

Thank you.

[Your Name]

Protecting Your Child from Nutrition and Health Education

With the increased national attention on children and weight, your child will likely hear food messages from authority figures in schools, day cares, and religious institutions, such as, "Enjoy your food, just eat less of it" printed on children's lunch menus. These can be confusing messages for all children, but especially to one who already eats little. There are reports that school nutrition education focused on calories and weight has triggered eating disorders (Pinhas et al. 2013), and parents are devastated when a child rejects a formerly safe food because lunchroom staff declared it unhealthy in front of the child's peers. A preemptive discussion with your child's teachers and principal is probably in order. Ask that your child not be weighed in school; many states mandate BMI testing in schools, and you may need to opt out in writing. Ask about the nutrition curriculum, and speak out if it focuses on labeling foods as "good" and "bad," or on calories and fat grams.

Talk to your child directly when you see or hear confusing messages she's exposed to. For example, if a visiting dental hygienist tells her class that juice, sugared cereals, and even fruit (which may include your child's safe foods) are unhealthy, say, **"Yes, if you ate those foods all day long and didn't brush your teeth it would be bad for your teeth. You don't need to worry about that."** Or **"Cake isn't bad—it's delicious. There are so many wonderful foods; your teacher is wrong on this one."** Remember, we believe no foods should be declared off limits or "bad." Check out the books at your child's preschool or day care. Many have messages about "good" and "bad" foods. Bring up concerns and offer to replace such books.

Finally, give your child's teacher the handout "How to Talk to Kids About Food" (online at http://www.newharbinger.com/31106). It provides ways to discuss food that stress joy and balance rather than increasing anxiety.

We can't protect our children from all pressure (especially living in a culture that doesn't generally support the idea of internally regulated eating), and it may be hard to stop counting calories, block out ignorant comments, or stand up to a beloved but pressuring teacher. What happens in your own home matters most, so first and foremost, keep hold of the DOR—the division of responsibility. Staying with your roles (the what, where, and when of feeding) and allowing your child his roles (the whether and how much of eating) will steer you away from power struggles, anxiety, and pressure. With time, the DOR and the steps in this chapter and the next four will be your new normal, as will enjoyment and peace at the table, and you'll look back with relief at the old, fading wagon-wheel ruts you, your child, and the rest of your family have left behind.

CHAPTER 5

Step 2: Establish a Structured Routine

In the last chapter, we learned how pressure and anxiety decrease appetite. While pressure is an obviously counterproductive tactic, other feeding practices may also undermine your child's eating. For example, Mary let her daughter, Lisa, watch TV with a bowl of ice cream every day to unwind after school, which meant Lisa wasn't hungry for dinner an hour later. Another mom, Clarice, so badly wanted "happy time" with her son Alex after a long day apart that she let him eat whatever and whenever he wanted. In addition to dictating TV and bedtime, Alex was eating fewer foods. Both mothers were stuck in counterproductive feeding, largely from a lack of structure.

We all have routines, whether we follow them by the clock or by the seat of our pants. Consider this—you always put your keys in the same place so you can grab them quickly in the morning. But one evening your teenager takes your car and leaves the keys elsewhere. What is your anxiety level during the fifteen-minute search? Routine and structure go hand in hand with reducing anxiety and getting through your day as smoothly as possible. In feeding, predictable meals and snacks are the steadying force—the scaffolding, if you will—that allows the other steps to succeed.

This chapter will help you establish and refine your feeding routine. Transitioning to structured eating opportunities is probably the single most important thing you can do to help your child tune in to appetite and eat well. A recent review of research found three additional key benefits: "increased parental efficacy, behavior monitoring, and coherence of family relationships" (Spagnola and Fiese 2007). So routines help children eat better, help you parent more effectively, and bring families closer together. Powerful stuff!

Understanding Appetite

Appetite is incredibly complex, but simply stated, it relates to how appealing a food is, or how much we look forward to eating it. Hunger is one component of appetite, but pure hunger is a physical need for fuel (and is also complex). Appetite, meanwhile, is affected by countless factors, from physiological (hormones, brain chemicals, stretch receptors in the stomach) to emotional (Grandma's apple pie) to experiential (negative experiences like choking). Appetite also involves how a food looks and smells, your mood, how long ago you last ate, whether you're on a diet (or have dieted before), and your temperament.

Your child can satisfy both hunger *and* appetite with appealing foods at the table and control over what goes in his mouth, eventually leading to healthy self-regulation and improved intake.

Exercise: If you eat on a regular schedule, delay eating your lunch for two hours. Do you feel anxious or tired? Another day, eat lunch much earlier than usual. How does it feel to eat when you aren't hungry? What do you notice when you look at your child's routine, the timing of meals, and his behavior?

How does your mealtime routine (or lack thereof) affect how you function and feel throughout the day? In other words, what is your *food and appetite temperament*? Are you ravenous in the morning, or can you skip breakfast and feel fine until lunch? We (Katja and Jenny) both have husbands who can go without eating all day, whereas we both eat regularly—or we get crabby and headachy! If you can comfortably skip meals, you may have a hard time understanding why your preschooler melts down midafternoon, and it may be harder for you to prioritize meals and snacks. We sometimes use the term "eating opportunity," which we have seen in various sources, instead of "meals and snacks." This term underlines the idea that meals and snacks are opportunities for your child to tune in to her appetite and explore foods, and for you to connect and observe her reactions and appetites.

Mismatched temperaments are challenging, but knowing that some people (possibly your child) feel poorly when hungry helps you empathize and prioritize eating opportunities. On the other hand, if you really enjoy and are tuned in to food, you may feel confused or hurt if your child doesn't share your pleasure. You may have to let go of your fantasies of baking Grandma's cookies together or bonding over sushi. It's okay to grieve that it isn't happening with your child right now, but find other things you love and can share.

Exercise: Go shopping when you are full and, another time, when famished. What do you notice about what looks appealing and what and how much you buy? How might this relate to your child's eating?

Grazing Dulls Appetite

Without routine, if your child sips and nibbles throughout the day (*grazing*), he will always have a little food, milk, or PediaSure in his tummy. Grazing sabotages hunger; your child may never feel hunger or learn that the hunger sensation in his stomach disappears when he eats.

Parents may report, "My child is never hungry," or, "He doesn't care about food." While it's true that some children are less driven by food, and some have medical or gastrointestinal issues (reflux, constipation, pain, bowel or stomach problems) that confuse or get in the way of appetite, almost all children can learn to recognize hunger. This is true even for the majority of those we have seen labeled "failure to thrive" or with feeding tubes and complex histories. Provided with regular meals and snacks, children have the *opportunity* to develop an appetite, maybe for the first time, and are more likely to eat to fullness.

Eating to fullness is contrasted with "taking the edge off" hunger by eating small amounts, which is the typical pattern for children who graze. When the stomach is comfortably full, special nerves called stretch receptors are stimulated, and the brain and body decrease hunger signals. With grazing, your child digests small amounts almost continuously, and may never experience the sensation of comfortable stretching. On the other hand, some children have a smaller stomach capacity from years of grazing or tube feeds, and an initial increase in volume may cause discomfort and, possibly, vomiting. Don't be surprised if your child's appetite only increases slowly, over time. Remember from our discussion on intake that appetite, quantity, and eating to fullness will vary from child to child and meal to meal.

Routine to the Rescue

If you have ever seen the TV shows *Supernanny* or *Nanny 911*, you'll notice they begin with the nanny making a schedule. Whether there is one child or half a dozen, routine is the cornerstone for the miraculous transformations you see in one hour of "reality" TV. While miracles may not happen in one hour in real life, routine helps behavior, anxiety, and appetite.

Routine Helps Behavior

We've all seen or *had* that child having a public meltdown, or dealt with the tween who storms off, slamming doors as she goes.

Children can lose control when they are off-kilter: tired, bored, hot, or over- or understimulated. Some children also struggle with transitions. Hunger or low blood sugar can make kids feel "off" too. But if your child isn't yet in touch with his hunger signals, or doesn't know how to communicate his hunger, you may assume that he is just behaving badly. Routine eating opportunities that offer fat or protein and carbohydrates (more on this later) help behavior by keeping a child's blood sugar levels stable, reducing spikes and crashes, and boosting attention and overall energy. Routine also promotes improved and longer sleep. Even an extra half hour of sleep can improve behavior and lessen hyperactivity.

Routine Helps Anxiety and Appetite

In general, children do best with routine—and even crave it—because of the inherent sense of stability. Many parents of children with sensory or anxiety concerns know that routine helps them manage strong input and emotions. Children better understand *what is expected of them when they know what to expect.* Routine and predictable meals meet a child's need for stability and can strengthen emotional connections. At mealtime, your child might talk about what she did that day or will do tomorrow. Rather than worry about when or where meals are and what rules apply, structure allows her to redirect her brainpower to looking at, exploring, or eating unfamiliar foods. Freeing her from worry supports appetite.

If grazing has knocked out your child's appetite, she'll be less interested in what's on the table. As the saying goes, "Hunger is the best cook" (or "sauce"). If your child comes to the table a little hungry, food is more appealing. And waiting *too long* between eating opportunities can harm appetite as much as grazing. If your child gets beyond ravenous, her appetite cues may disappear or be hard to interpret. Have you ever noticed that if you don't eat during a window of hunger, you might not feel like yourself, or you might get a headache, but you don't necessarily feel hungry?

Routine Makes Molehills out of Mountains

Feeding your child with EPE can feel like climbing a mountain without ever reaching the top. When you think you're almost there, a new feeding stage pops up, or your child gets sick, has a bad day at school, or didn't take that nap he needed, and you feel like you are losing ground. With structured routine, bumps in the road don't become mountains. Your child trusts that he will have another opportunity to eat soon, and that not eating well at dinner for whatever reason isn't the end of the world—for you or for him. You can go about your bedtime routine, knowing that he might eat a larger breakfast than normal. And after a bad day at school, your child can rely on a predictable snack or dinnertime to restore his equilibrium.

Transitioning to a Routine of Sit-Down Meals and Snacks

This section explores strategies to transition to and support routine meals and snacks. Your child's personality and flexibility will determine what kinds of support she needs, and how much. Paired with these strategies are *routine-building activities*, which we do to prepare children for what comes next. Note that if meals and snacks are currently hit-or-miss, you should start on a weekend, or when things will be calmer than usual. As with potty training or moving to a big-kid bed, extra time at the beginning gives you and your child wiggle room if things don't go so well at first.

Treating Meals and Snacks Equally

Many parents view "meals" and "snacks" differently, in terms of what is offered and how: snacks are often one item, intended to hold a child over until the meal. But, the traditional snack time (after school) may be when your child is hungriest, and offering balanced choices and enough so that he may eat to fullness is ideal. The word "meal" may also spike anxiety if meals have been marked by conflict. Thinking of meals and snacks as four or five equivalent daily *opportunities for eating* opens the door for change.

Food for Thought: In your journal, write down the words "Breakfast," "Snack," "Lunch," "Snack," and "Dinner." Assign approximate starting and finishing times based on your family's schedule. Do times change on different days? What activities or issues keep you from sticking to these times? (More on timing in the section "Flexibility in Routine" later in this chapter.)

Supporting Routine

Some studies suggest that it takes about two weeks for a new habit to become ingrained. With busy schedules, it may take several weeks before your routine feels natural, and even the most regular routine can still feel hectic. Simplify where you can: do you have to volunteer at Meals on Wheels right now? Does your son need to be in two sports? One mom we know limits each of her three children to one extracurricular activity at a time and makes family meals a top priority—at least as important as playing an instrument. Learning to eat is a life skill worthy of the commitment. Take your time establishing a routine, and expect it to feel challenging at first. Even if you, personally, feel constricted by routines, keep in mind that structure is critical to success. Flexibility, addressed later, is possible within an overall consistent structure. To support routine:

- Use natural breaks in your child's day to build in snacks: after a nap or school, or before karate.

- Explore family calendar apps, or get a large calendar for the wall or desktop to track activities and a general menu. This helps avoid the "what's for dinner?" scramble that trips up routine (we offer meal-planning tips in chapter 7).

- Try a dry-erase board for menu and routine planning. Kids can decorate it to look like a fancy restaurant menu, and you can easily erase and adjust.

- Plan for about two to three hours between eating opportunities for younger children, or about three to four hours for children kindergarten-age and older.

- On busy days, think creatively about timing. Katja used to pick her daughter up from preschool and they would sit in the parked car and eat; if her daughter ate in a moving car, she was distracted and didn't eat to fullness, but the drive home was too long to wait. You may find it helps to stop by a park and eat, or go into the restaurant rather than use the drive-through.

- Invest in an insulated bag and icepack to transport snacks and keep things fresh.

- If your child takes medications, supplements, or vitamins, and you are good about giving them, this routine can support a mealtime routine: plan meals to coincide.

Minimize Distractions

With a low appetite, distractions (in various forms) are often more interesting than the food. Minimize distractions to support routine: change the seating arrangement (so little brother can't poke your child with EPE), remove pets during meals, and ask others to leave gadgets and reading in another room. Chapter 8 addresses how to wean your family off any distractions you may have come to rely on.

Managing Transitions

If your child is sensitive, anxious, or very active, likes things to be his idea, or needs to feel in control, he may struggle with transitions.

If he is old enough, talk to him about your new routine so he knows what to expect; you could say something like **"We want to have a better time at the table, so we're doing things a little differently. We'll all come to the table for meals, and we'll let you know when it's time to get ready."** Mary, whose son was working with a therapist for anxiety, found that specific help around transitions supported routine and appetite tremendously; for example, **"In five minutes, we'll stop for snack (put away toys, wash hands)."** Or **"In five minutes, we'll wash hands and you can put out the napkins and silverware."**

You may find that calming music prepares your child for meals. For children with sensory integration challenges, feeding therapist Suzanne Evans Morris recommends Hemi-Sync (Hemispheric Synchronization) music—music with audio patterns that promote brainwave synchronization. "Children and adults," she writes, "often become less anxious and more open to new possibilities when listening to recordings containing Hemi-Sync" (Morris 2002, 2). In her paper "User's Guide: Hemi-Sync for Learning and Stress Reduction," Morris recommends particular recordings that increase focus and deepen relaxation.

If your child has difficulty staying engaged with activities or is coming to the table directly after sleeping, he may need to alert his body that it's time to eat. Plan high-energy activities such as trampoline jumping or a quick tickle session before meals to "get the wiggles out" so he can attend to what's on the table.

Involving your child in appropriate meal and table preparation keeps her busy and makes her feel competent, important, and part of the family—and helps you! You might say **"I need your help washing the potatoes, and you're so good at it!"** Children who help prepare foods *are more likely* to try them, but there's no guarantee. Generally, noting the positive works better than stern reminders, but a word of caution is in order: avoid positive feedback for *what* or *how much* your child eats. Say instead **"I like how you're putting your toys away."** Or **"Good job finding your apron!"**

If your child needs more transition time or reminders, find what works for you. A cleanup song supports routine through ritual and music, while a wall chart reminds visual learners what's next. Try printing pictures of your child doing different tasks and make a schedule board; some children get a sense of accomplishment from task cards with Velcro that they move to the "done" side. Older children feel more grown-up and respected if they help make the schedule: for example, they might choose whether homework comes before or after dinner. Tweens using technology might find that an electronic day planner is more empowering than reminders from Mom or Dad!

In considering when and why your routine falls apart, you may find that the pestering child is the biggest barrier to getting the sweet potato fries out of the oven. The temptation to allow your son to nibble on appetite-killing pretzels to keep him out of the way may be too much if you're not prepared (note this differs from the "tide-me-over" discussed later in the chapter). Here are some ideas to keep children busy while you get food on the table:

- Have them do homework at the kitchen island or table while you prep: they can ask for help, and you have company.

- Put them to work—laying the table, feeding the dog, or emptying the dishwasher. Jenny's sons know that when they get home, Mom starts dinner, and they unload the dishwasher. Very young children can sort cups or put out napkins or spoons.

- Toddlers may enjoy a drawer or shelf with Tupperware or pots to play with.

- Fill a shallow bin with dry oats or rice and let children scoop, measure, and play.

- Put together a box of special toys, art supplies, games, or activity books to be used while you prepare the meal.

- Use screen time (if your family allows it) to your advantage—maybe allow video games or cartoons for fifteen minutes before dinner.

New routines and transitions take time and effort on your part initially, but as everyone gets used to the predictable structure, the decrease in conflict, whining and uncertainty is worth the investment.

Flexibility in Routine

Some parents bristle at the idea of routine, particularly parents who are laid-back or have a temperament that allows them to comfortably skip meals. But routines can be flexible, and they need to work for your family, not the other way around. If you keep the general time frame and the idea of "eating opportunities" in mind, it can lessen resentment toward the clock. You might have several different routines: one for weekends where you sleep in; another for softball nights or when you work late; another to anticipate changes like vacations, your youngest dropping naps, and so on.

In general, offer food every two to three hours to children kindergarten-age and younger, and to older children every three to four hours. You don't need to wake a napping child to eat or offer a midmorning snack if breakfast and lunch are close enough together. Keeping the time range in mind is the key. Initially, try to have as regular a routine as possible, and introduce flexibility as you all get the hang of it. (For children weaning from feeding tubes, your dietitian should help with the schedule to optimize appetite and nutrition.) Here are some tips for making routines flexible:

- If your child comes home starving after school or day care, serve "dinner" then. Provide a balanced offering, and plan another eating opportunity again two to four hours later—a late-working partner can enjoy her or his meal at that time so you can eat together.

- Move dinner or snack up by half an hour. No need to tell your child you are doing it or why; just do it.

- If there is a playdate with the usual carbohydrate buffet and it's not meal or snack time, you have options. If you are new to STEPS+ and want to stick with the routine, you can skip the playdate for now, *or* plan playdates at eating times, *or* recognize that the occasional playdate where your child eats and spoils his appetite is fine. He might not eat much the next time he sits down to eat, but routine means he'll have another chance in a few hours.

- Let it go on special days: Friday nights with grandparents, school picnics, or cookies after a religious service.

Sometimes, children *are* really hungry but dinner isn't ready, or you got home late, or snack happened somewhere distracting. If you don't want to or can't adjust mealtime, offer a *tide-me-over*. Unlike the planned snack where your child eats until full, this is a little food to hold him over until the meal. It might be frozen peas, cut up cucumber, a few crackers, or a small amount of a safe food. If there has been a lot of mealtime stress, a tide-me-over may feel like a safe space for him to branch out, so consider including a new food. It is fine to serve a tide-me-over at a different spot than the regular mealtime table (such as a child-size table or coffee table). Here is some language to try with a tide-me-over:

"Would you like frozen peas or carrots and ranch* for your tide-me-over?"

"Here's a tide-me-over—we'll save some hungry for dinner."

"Get yourself a small bowl of crackers; dinner will be soon."

"Here are some grapes; then you can help set the table."

* "Wait," you might think, "Isn't it *my job* to decide what she eats?" In time, you can allow your child to make some decisions about what is offered at meals and snacks, as she is capable. (More about this in chapter 7.)

When Your Child Tests the Routine

As with any change, children may resist (some more than others), testing to see if you plan to stick with the change. They may test how far they can push the limits by resisting sitting at the table, not eating anything, or acting out. Be clear about your expectations, saying, for example: **"We sit together for dinner. I know we haven't always done this, but we are starting tonight."** Or **"We like your company at dinnertime. Sit with us for a few minutes and tell us about your day. You don't have to eat anything you don't want to."**

If your child won't come to the table, consider if he still feels anxious there: are you arguing about manners, preplating meals, praising him for bites, or insisting he drink his smoothie? Kids avoid a table with pressure. Some parents find success using a kitchen timer, saying something like: **"You don't have to eat anything, but we love your company. Can you set this timer for five minutes? When the timer runs out, you can stay, or you may go and play quietly so we can finish our dinner."** Make pleasant conversation, have a place set for your child, avoid pressure, and let him leave if he wants at the end of the five minutes. We have observed that rather quickly, if the table is a pleasant place, he'll want to stay and even start eating. Limiting the time initially can reassure an anxious child.

When He Won't Eat Anything

In the past when your child refused to eat, during meals you may have allowed him to fetch a favorite food just so he ate *something*. With your new routine, and the rest of the steps—and where the eating opportunity is pressure-free and includes at least one safe choice—you won't let him get up and get crackers. Be prepared for your child to test you, not eating much, if anything, for a meal or two to see if he can wait you out and get what he wants.

To help preserve your sanity and ease your child into the routine, you might at first provide two foods he can eat, providing only one later as he learns the routine. Try not to worry about each mealtime, but look for change over a day or week. If your child eats *nothing at all* for more than a few meals in a row, *and* you are providing safe choices, contact your child's health care team.

Apply the above ideas when your child won't eat at mealtimes, but if he chooses not to eat and comes back soon after the meal asking for his favorite, calmly remind him of the new routine. You might say: **"Lunch is over. Snack is soon—let's go play a game."** Or **"I'm sorry, sweetie; dinner is over. I'll start the bath; you pick a book for after."**

If he's used to getting food when he wants and he knows you worry, this is one of the hardest habits to change. Accepting a new routine usually takes a few days to a week, but if you stick with it, he will realize there will be a chance to eat, including a safe food, every two to four hours (depending on his age) and he will be less motivated to resist and test you. Routine is your safety net.

If you anticipate your child refusing to eat, you could serve dinner earlier to allow time for a bedtime snack. Ellyn Satter calls this the "rescue snack," a fitting name. If your child is offered accepted foods before bed, you'll be more comfortable letting her eat less at dinner and less likely to allow her to pick different foods than you offered.

If feeding is severely strained or your child is very anxious, start with an easy bedtime snack, maybe even a small candy or sweet (see chapter 7). When meals were very stressful for one family, Jenny suggested they offer cereal in a cup on the beanbag chair during bedtime stories, to help the child feel safe while eating *something*. The dad shared, "We did this early on while Corbin was learning to self-feed and be less terrified of food; it helped him realize that food can be looked forward to and enjoyed."

What If My Child Can't Sit?

Some children wander or play during meals. You may have even been encouraged to allow it, as a way to "get more food in," but like other distractions, wandering decreases intake overall. Many mothers share this frustration: "He'll leave the table, saying he's done, and when I take away his plate, he screams for it. Then he sits there pushing the food around but doesn't eat."

Give a warning, such as **"If you leave the table again, it tells me you are done and I'll put your plate away."** When he leaves, put away his plate. If he then wants it back, calmly remind him of the new expectations. Usually it takes only a handful of times for your child to understand the new rules. If you slip up and give the plate back sometimes, it's not the end of the world, but it might confuse your child, and he might push harder next time. If he doesn't eat anything, remember the bedtime snack option discussed above.

If you think your child can't sit because he is fidgety or needs more movement, plan physical activities during the day or before mealtime—dancing, mini trampoline, Wii games, and so on. Make sure his seat has a sturdy footrest, as dangling feet are distracting. Sensory seekers may have a hard time sitting still; one boy Jenny worked with would stand and eat happily at the table while bouncing on his toes. You might also place an inflatable sensory cushion in his seat for more input to help him focus.

> **Food for Thought:** If you're feeling annoyed or pulled into a power struggle, pause before you react. Is your child pushing the limits of the routine, or taking over your job of deciding what foods are offered? Or is his behavior part of his sensory reality or need for predictability? Can you accommodate his needs as he transitions to the new way of eating, like the mom who enjoyed meals with her son standing at the table?

Not sitting is common, especially if tuning in to appetite is new. Trust your gut. One mother shared that her four-year-old who grazed and never once asked for food would happily eat a small amount at the beginning of dinner, and then say he was done. She didn't pressure him to eat and allowed him to play quietly close by while she and his dad ate. Occasionally, as they were transitioning to routine, he would come back and eat more, and Mom wondered if that was okay. She sensed it was helping him tune in to hunger and fullness signals since he was eating more during his time at the table, and, importantly, everyone was happier and less stressed.

Some experts would have said not to let him back; he'll throw a tantrum and that's that. That works for many families, and is often advice we've given, depending on the situation. However, if your child is not disrupting, and your motivation for allowing him to play is not about getting in two more bites, he may use this time to observe you and listen to his body as he learns how much to eat to feel full. This is often a transitional step on the way to sitting through a whole meal, especially if meals have been stressful. You can learn to tell the difference between the process of tuning in and a power play.

When Your Child Acts Out at Meals

Although mealtime behavior usually improves with STEPS+, your child might—as with other changes in her life—push back by acting out. Your child's personality and temperament play a big part in her reaction. If she does act out, start by asking yourself how you would handle things if you weren't at the table. Use techniques that work for you. If time-outs work well at other times, use them at eating opportunities. If warnings or "time-ins" work best, use those. If you are struggling to find a way to help your child deal with big feelings or behavior, find help. Here are some ideas of what to say if she needs a break from the table to calm down.

"We want to have a good time at lunch, but it isn't nice when you are screaming (kicking, throwing food, and so on). You can come back when you can be pleasant."

"We'll go to your room for a time-out and come back when you are ready."

"When you're ready to be with us again, we'll be waiting with hugs." (From Dawn Friedman, writer and family therapist, on her blog *Building Family Counseling*.)

If she doesn't come back during the meal, routine means you can hold firm and not give her food ten minutes after the table is cleared.

While most children feel relief and blossom when they are no longer the mealtime focus, others may grieve the loss of attention, even if it was mostly negative. When you stop hovering and prompting bites, your child may act out or regress in other areas like potty training or bedtime. If a big part of your child's identity is being the "picky" eater, she'll have to figure out who she is apart from that. You can help her work through her loss if you realize it's happening. Do a puzzle or color together after or before meals, or watch funny animal videos—laugh, have fun, and help her get to know herself without food in the equation.

Routine Is Here to Stay

If you stick with these changes and make sure that others at your table (siblings, grandparents) are aware of them, your child will realize routine is here to stay. This doesn't mean you become a drill sergeant; rather, your consistent, simple, and calm explanations of what is going to happen and when will help her adapt—again, children do better when they know what to expect. After a week or so of pressure-free opportunities to see how it all works, things should start to settle. Even tweens not used to family meals eventually look forward to that time together if it's about connection and respect. They might sulk at first, or complain that family dinners are "lame," but don't let them talk you out of it!

When Structure Isn't Really Structure

Four-year-old Nathan ate fewer than ten foods, "failed" twelve months of behavioral and sensory therapies, and was at the first percentile for weight. His mom, Elise, thought she had a routine—and she and Nathan did have a *rhythm* to their days. However, a common problem emerged when she wrote down when eating started and ended:

6:30–7:00 a.m.: sippy of milk—Nathan enjoys cuddle time in bed with mother, father, and baby sister, who gets a bottle at the same time

8–9:15 a.m.: at the table for breakfast

10–11:30 a.m.: snack (crackers while wandering around)

12–1:30 p.m.: lunch

3–4:00 p.m.: snack (crackers while playing)

5–6:45 p.m.: dinner

Did you catch it? They spent far too long (six hours a day) at the table or with food, hoping Nathan would eat a few more bites. With an hour or less between eating opportunities and a little something in his tummy most of the day, he had no chance to develop an appetite. The "routine" *turned into grazing.* This pattern is all too common, but it is full of opportunities for progress—starting with the morning sippy cup. Many families rely on supplements or milk for nutrition, often giving a sippy cup or bottle first thing with a cuddle. When told to "get rid of" a bottle or sippy cup for an older child, parents report upset children whose intake drops dramatically. To phase out the sippy or bottle while supporting appetite, try these suggestions:

- Continue the cuddle or special time, and bring the milk or bottle into routine meals. Say: **"Mommy loves our morning cuddle, and now that you're four, we'll cuddle and read, and we'll have our milk at breakfast."**

- Use natural opportunities for change, like a new daycare provider, or starting kindergarten. Say: **"You'll start first grade at the end of the summer. Let's practice being a first-grader and have your milk with breakfast. Let's read together in the morning."**

Many families are pleasantly surprised that within a few days the kids are used to the new routine: they are attached to cuddle time, not the sippy! It supports the child's appetite *and* emotional needs to bring the sippy or bottle into the routine, phasing it out rather than going cold turkey.

These changes helped Nathan and his family get on track. Another tip to optimize appetite is to set an approximate time limit on meals and snacks. Ideally, Nathan needs at least two hours between the end of one eating opportunity and the beginning of the next. Within a few days of Mom shortening the time at the table, and removing pressure, Nathan ate a larger than usual breakfast and even said "I'm hungry" for the first time!

Generally, we suggest an upper limit of about thirty to forty minutes for meals, and twenty to thirty minutes for snacks. Sometimes, children are anxious about ending meals. Having something to look forward to usually helps. When limiting mealtime, you might say something like: **"In about five minutes we're going to play with Legos (or draw, or listen to music)."** Or **"In ten minutes we'll get ready for bed—your new book is waiting!"**

The Skittish Appetite

Learning to tune in to hunger is a developmental skill. If your child is behind with this skill, it will take her time to figure out if she is hungry or what those sensations feel like. She, for whatever reason, may never have had this opportunity, or else she may have been confused by other feelings, such as pain from ongoing or past reflux. Early appetite signals can be skittish and unsure, and any pressure can make them go away. As parents mull over routines and limiting time at the table, we often hear, "What should I do if he ever *does* say he's hungry, but it's not time to eat? I can't imagine not giving him food if he asks."

Skye Van Zetten, blogging at *Mealtime Hostage,* once shared her approach with her son, TJ, who has food anxiety and EPE. One morning at the grocery store, he asked to try some strawberry fruit leather (the first time he asked to try a food). Skye calmly opened the package and handed it to him. He tried it—and liked it! Even though it wasn't "time" to eat, he expressed an interest (showing internal motivation) and was not being manipulative—that is, Mom did not feel like he was trying to get out of his usual mealtimes. Also, TJ had a history of easily getting upset and losing his appetite completely. Skye usually stuck with the routine, which was helping, but she felt she chose well in this situation. The bottom line is that you can trust your instincts and what you know about your child. Don't worry if you don't completely trust your instincts yet. The STEPS+ approach will help you observe how your child reacts and gain confidence in your ability to anticipate his needs and respond in supportive ways.

Consistent but flexible routine, with meals and snacks as equivalent eating opportunities offered without pressure, gives you, your child, and your family needed structure and stability. With routine, you help your child decrease anxiety and increase appetite. You'll support his internal motivation to learn to eat more foods while you enjoy enough flexibility to respond in loving ways that meet your need to nurture. (Your needs matter too!)

In the next chapter we'll talk about step 3—family meals. You'll learn where to start and how to make your table a welcoming place, even for the most skittish appetites.

CHAPTER 6

Step 3: Have Family Meals

Several studies (including Andaya et al. 2011) have found that family meals (including breakfast, lunch and dinner) predict success in life and are linked to better nutrition, more stable weight, and less risk of developing an eating disorder. Family meals are a time to pass on family stories, traditions, and culture—and to laugh and spend enjoyable time with your children away from work, homework, and other distractions. The family meal becomes a dependable anchor for the family.

Making family meals a priority is tough, what with after-school activities, extended workdays, time to shop, or not knowing how to prepare quick, balanced, and tasty meals. According to a 2013 Gallup poll, only about half of Americans regularly sit down to family meals. Forty percent of parents in one study prepared separate meals for their grade school–aged children (Fulkerson et al. 2008), a percentage we predict would be even higher for families impacted by extreme picky eating. Parents give up on family meals if everyone is generally happier *without* them.

We hear most often that dinner is the trickiest meal. More challenging foods are often served, and homework, fatigue and bedtime loom. But dinner *can* go from the worst to one of the best parts of your day. An African proverb says "When the music changes, so does the dance." This chapter is about changing the music. If meals are a place of connection and joy, the effort is worthwhile and sustainable.

Here you'll find a smorgasbord of ideas to get you started on feel-good family meals: what to say, how to model manners, where and how to offer foods, and more.

What Is a Family Meal?

Parents come to the table with ideas about what family meals are or should be. Many adults didn't eat meals with their own parents and can't picture a pleasant family meal. One father shared that his child-hood dinners were somber. He wanted more *fun* with his children, and so he resisted eating together around a table.

> **Food for Thought:** What do you remember about meals as a child? How much of your memories are about *the food*? Imagine the ideal meal with *your* children. What is it like?

A family meal is, at its most basic, members of a family (with one or more loving adults) sitting with the children and eating at the same time, from the same foods, without significant distractions. "Family meals" include breakfast, lunch, dinner, *and* snacks. Sitting with your child with a cup of coffee or tea while she eats her snack can turn snack time into a family meal. Ideally, especially early on, make every eating opportunity at home a family meal—an opportunity to connect and model around food. *You* are the most important thing at the table, not the vegetables. Studies suggest that a big part of what helps young children learn what is good to eat is watching adults they trust. Free from having to negotiate or enforce bites or portion mini-mums, you too can enjoy family meals. As one mom said, "I don't have anxiety attacks before dinner anymore!" Once you are sitting down to the meal, your role is to create a pleasant atmosphere and:

- Model manners: "Please," "thank you," or "no thank you."

- Enjoy foods you enjoy. Talk positively or in a neutral way about all foods. Remember the phrase "Don't yuck my yum." Don't fake loving a food. Don't say "yuck" or "gross" either. *You* get to say, "No thank you."

- Save stressful topics or arguing for another time and place.

- Pick your battles. Let bad manners or chewing with an open mouth go for now.

- Enjoy playful moments—as long as silliness is not used as a distraction to get more food in.

Your child, used to being the focus at meals, must be allowed to just be a *participant*. A former selective eater seeking help for his daughter's eating described his experience this way: "I can pinpoint the meal where it changed. I was ten. My parents had given up on my eating, with no nagging, bribing, or discussions for a while. I had the plain, boring stuff I always ate, and my parents had Chinese food. I remember the good smells and thinking, 'That looks way better than mine.' So I tried and liked some. By the end of summer I was eating ten times more foods than before."

This story illustrates the importance of a child's being allowed to be part of a family meal (not the focus) without pressure, so that internal motivation ("I want some!") and curiosity have room to grow. The former selective eater's parents gave up on making him eat, but not on family meals!

Family Table Mood Makeover

If the table is a stressful place, a "makeover" signals that things will be different. This can involve new plates or placemats, having your child make a centerpiece, even moving to a different table or hanging new curtains. If Dad is bothered by Lucy eating with her mouth open, or Mom is arguing with Max about manners, switch the seating: have Dad sit next to, not directly across from, Lucy; and have Mom do the same with Max. If your child is in a highchair with a tray, remove the tray if she's able—nothing says "I'm part of the family meal" like being pulled right up to the table.

Consider Obstacles

What are some of the obstacles to making family meals happen? Think of creative ways to get around them. For example:

- High, bar stool–height table and chairs: Replace with standard table and chairs.

- No dishwasher: Use plastic or paper plates.

- Small table: Place serving bowls on a card table, TV stand, or nearby bookshelf. Use smaller serving bowls and refill.

- No kitchen table: Add stools at the island so you can eat together, make space for a kitchen table, or convert a closet into office space to free up the dining room table.

- Carpeting, or fear of mess: Remove carpeting from eating areas or cover with a plastic sheet or old rug. Mess is unavoidable. Keep a small vacuum handy for cleanup.

If the table triggers anxiety, you might start with picnics around the coffee table, or blankets on the floor. If you eat together, even if it's take-out served at the coffee table, it's a family meal. You might play a favorite game at the family table, with a favorite snack or no food at all. Let your child win! The goal is to begin associating good feelings with a formerly stressful place (more in chapter 8). If dinner is most stressful, start with breakfast or brunch.

Consider Your Child's Sensory Temperament

Think about your child's sensory temperament (explored in chapter 2). Simplify mealtime, and limit distractions as much as you can if your child is easily overwhelmed: get white plates and solid-colored, thicker placemats to deaden sounds; turn off the television or loud music.

Exercise: Get on your child's level and think about his sensory experiences: look at the lighting and think about what he hears, how the silverware feels, if table legs are in the way, and other possible distractions.

Get Centered Before Meals

Pause to connect before you eat: say a grace (religious or not), thank the cook, maybe hold hands, sing a song, light a candle—LED without flame for younger children—and let the kids blow it out. Start the meal calm and tuned in, rather than ready for battle.

Serve Foods Family (Buffet) Style

If you preplate your child's meals with what and how much you want her to eat, the battle probably begins before the plate hits the table: "I don't like that!" "It's touching!" "How much do I have to eat?" Your child's focus is on the negotiation, and her appetite plummets.

Serving family style sounds intimidating, but it simply means putting the food in the middle of the table so everyone can serve themselves. *Serving meals family style is the number one thing parents say defuses battles at the table.* As Skye Van Zetten observed of her son, "Once he was given the option to choose what he wanted on his plate and permission to do with it whatever he wanted, family meals immediately took a turn for the better." Here are some tips for serving family style:

- Put out a bowl of your child's safe food with the other foods—even if it seems silly to put the applesauce in the middle of the table.

- Forget fancy serving ware. Use sturdy, dishwasher-safe stackable glass or plastic serving bowls.

- Use trivets and bring the casserole, pan, or pot to the table if you don't feel like washing another bowl. Help children if there are hot pans on the table.

- Put take-out containers in the middle of the table.

- Set out accepted condiments with every meal: a bottle of ketchup, hot sauce, butter, and so on.

- Consider using a lazy Susan for serving dishes.

- Present all foods the same way, from broccoli to crackers, with no more "kid" and "grown-up" foods or "yours" or "mine."

Even if your child only eats crackers or noodles (for now), you are erasing the separations—part of what made your child the focus. Now it's *just dinner,* and you all choose from what's available.

Helping Children Serve Themselves

To the extent that your child is able, allow him to serve himself from what's on the table. For more difficult foods like soup, or if your child is still learning or has developmental delays, you can help serve him in ways that give him some control, such as guiding his hand with the serving spoon, or doing every step with permission. Ask, for example, **"Would you like some mashed potatoes?"** If your child says yes, hold the spoon out with a small amount on it: **"This much?"** Adjust accordingly and check in. When he says yes, say, **"Point to where you would like it."**

With nonverbal or younger children, look for signs of permission before placing something on their plates or highchair trays. Occupational therapist and feeding expert Marsha Dunn Klein uses the image of the "positive tilt" in her work. Does the child give permission by tilting toward you and the food, or is she leaning back, signaling she's not ready?

When you serve family style, leave the serving plates within your child's reach so that when she is ready (usually when Mom and Dad are chatting with each other or a sibling) she can reach out and help herself (as you pretend you don't notice!). Sometimes this way of serving meals can even entice children to be more adventurous. If someone else (particularly a sibling) has something, many children, in an effort to keep everything "fair," want it too. We call this the "scarcity effect." One mom shared, "We noticed when I'd say, 'I'm going to finish the peas if no one minds,' he'd suddenly put some on his plate." She then asked, "Can we trick him into eating by doing this more often?" If you notice this "scarcity effect" at work, that's fine, but tread carefully. Chances are he'll figure out if you use it to trick him, and it will slow progress. Observe and be curious about his reactions to family-style meals.

Some therapists recommend including a "looking" or "tasting" plate of foods next to the child's plate. She is then asked to kiss, poke, or smell the foods on the plate. If your child likes this, you can try it. But she may react negatively if she feels pressured (that is, if anxiety, temperament, and past experiences come into play). The nice thing about family-style meals is that your child gets to see and smell different foods, pass a bowl, and, if she knows she can serve herself (or others) with no expectation to eat, lick, or kiss the food, explore in her own time.

Helping Her Feel Comfortable with Her Own Seat and Plate

Remember that part of learning to eat happens when children watch their parents eat. Many parents note that their child with EPE will eat from *their* plates but not his own. Why? This is partly because if it comes from Mom or Dad's plate, then it is safe. They *trust* you to keep them safe. While this developmental phase typically happens for older infants and young toddlers, your child may have some catching up to do.

Sometimes a child wants to eat sitting on a parent's lap. This can be the result of a child trying to keep parents' attention (in light of the loss of focus on his eating), or because Mom stops pressuring when the child is on Dad's lap. On your side, the temptation may be to allow her on your lap "to get more bites in," which can result in the five-year-old who only eats while being spoon-fed on a parent's lap.

If your anxious child has recently started climbing onto your lap or eating from your plate, you may decide during this transition to allow it occasionally, if it helps her feel safe and explore new foods. But be careful not to let it become the *only* way she eats. Here are tips to help your child be comfortable at her own place at the table:

- Build in a few minutes of closeness before or right after meals—cuddle with a book, or sing a song with her in your lap.

- Engage him in conversation and give positive attention during meals for specific things: **"You did such a nice job setting the table!"**

- Use your bowl as a temporary serving bowl. Spoon a few items from your plate, with permission, onto his.

One mom told Jenny how her son climbed onto her lap and used her crackers to dip into her soup—eating soup for the first time. Jenny suggested that Mom help her son spoon soup into his bowl from hers, so he knew it was the same. Then when he was happily eating, Mom would "forget" her napkin and get up to get it. Mom would then move him to his chair (close to hers) with his bowl as he kept eating. If the table is pleasant and free from pressure, such a transition has a higher chance of success.

Serve Dessert with the Rest of the Food

Our clients tell us that after serving family style, *serving dessert with the meal is the second most helpful tip*, though it's often the strategy that meets with the most resistance. Pause and register your reaction to the idea of allowing your child to eat dessert *with* dinner, even before anything else. Serving dessert *with* the meal feels threatening to many parents who worry that their child will eat *only* dessert—which he might for a time—or that without bribes, he won't eat anything "healthy." (As we've said previously, bribing with dessert doesn't help long-term, and we recommend not doing it.) Hang in there—it's part of the process.

To set the table with dessert, the main dish and sides go in the middle, and each place setting has an empty plate, perhaps a bowl for salad or a side dish, and a spot for dessert. Dessert may be a cookie on a napkin, or a serving of pudding, ice cream, or fruit in a bowl. Frozen desserts can stay in the freezer and come out when kids are ready. If children are able, tell them **"Your ice cream is ready for you in the fridge when you want it."** *Limit the dessert to one appropriate serving— and no seconds.* Unlimited desserts could lower your child's appetite and motivation to try other foods (Satter 2000).

Decisions about the type and amount of dessert depend on your child's age, how long since she last ate, and your guess about how much of the other food she will likely enjoy. A few tablespoons of ice cream, a small frozen fruit pop, or two small animal crackers might be appropriate for a child with a low appetite. A child with a larger appetite or one who has learned to tune in to signals from her body may get a larger cookie or half a cup of ice cream. If there is only one other safe food available, you might provide a larger serving of fruit for dessert to round out the meal.

With siblings, equal servings minimize arguments. You are in charge of what is presented for dinner, so once you decide what dessert will be, don't give in to requests for more. This is different than the planned treat snack (discussed in chapter 7) where you allow your child to eat as much as she likes of what is served.

Expect your child to eat dessert first for a time—anywhere from a few days to several weeks. The new dessert setup may confuse older children if dessert has been used as motivation to eat. Explain the new approach: **"We are going to start having dessert with dinner. You** can eat it whenever you want." Or **"None of us likes arguing over how many bites of food you have to eat to get dessert. So, we're doing things differently."**

When they ask how much of X they have to eat to get dessert, say **"You can eat the dessert first if you want."** Or **"Sounds like you're sad you can't have Popsicles for dessert** (*pause to acknowledge and allow an answer*). **We had them yesterday. We'll have them again soon."** Or **"That's your share. If you're still hungry you can have more X, Y, or Z."** Or **"I wish we could swim in a pool of pudding! Chocolate pudding hot tubs!"** Join in with fantasy talk to have some fun and defuse upset, as Adele Faber and Elaine Mazlish (2012) describe in *How to Talk So Kids Will Listen and Listen So Kids Will Talk*.

Many parents didn't grow up eating dessert, and would rather eat more of the main meal. It's okay if your child is the only one having dessert; or if she doesn't miss dessert, you don't have to serve it. However, if your child asks for it often because she's five (they tend to at that age), or if dessert is the overly prized forbidden food, we suggest including desserts or treats at meals and snacks, about once a day. Some parents find harmony when they allow their children to choose which meal or snack includes the daily dessert.

The Paper Napkin Security Blanket

Set the table with paper napkins so children can spit food out. Particularly for children with a history of gagging or vomiting, knowing they can get something out of their mouths *without* gagging or vomiting decreases anxiety, making them more willing to try new foods. Some children don't have the oral motor skills to spit food out yet. If your child sees a speech therapist, this is one of the first things she should help your child with. Young children can spit food out on the tray or table, over time learning to subtly spit food in the napkin so they can do this away from home.

> **Food for Thought:** Imagine that you, in a foreign country, are served a tan stew with unknown ingredients. Might you be more willing to try it if you could spit it out? (With no one pressuring or watching!) What if someone explained the flavors and you could explore it with a spoon as well?

Some parents think it's rude to spit food out. One local farming educator said he makes the grade-school children he visits swallow vegetable samples "out of respect for the farmer." We believe respecting the child's limits is more important than a notion of politeness or respect for the farmer or cook. Allowing children to (politely) spit out food is critical. Say: **"You have a paper napkin if you want to spit something out."**

Tell your child about the napkin once or twice, not several times each meal, which turns into pressure. Avoid, for example: "Don't forget, sweetie, if you want to try that, you can spit it out, remember?"

Offering Food the Better Way

Many parents believe they offer foods over and over, but here is what happens: Mom or Dad stands at the fridge or pantry throwing out suggestions. "You want pizza? How about spaghetti? Chicken? No? What do you want?" Even adventurous children can't be expected to decide the menu—that's your job. Truly offering in a way that doesn't immediately invite "no" means putting the foods out, preferably family style, so your child can choose: perhaps sweet potato fries, rolls, chicken breast, canned mandarin oranges, and broccolini broiled with Parmesan.

Don't Ask, Don't Tell

The hardest part is offering without encouraging, reminding, or pressuring. The more you say, the more your child will argue (many children are masterful negotiators):

"I made it the way you like it." (No you didn't, it's too chewy.)

"It's not too hot." (Yes it is!)

"I took off the cheese you don't like." (I don't like the sauce either.)

Also avoid the trap of asking questions your child can say no to, or that shut down exploration:

"Is it too hot?" (It is too hot. I'm not eating it!)

"You like this, don't you? You ate it yesterday." (No! I don't like it anymore!)

"Do you want two or three bites?" (None!)

"I don't think you like these, but do you want to try them?" (No way!)

Offer, Enjoy It Yourself, Wait, Repeat

A client who is also a dietitian tells of the summer with the bumper crop of raspberries. Every day her son joyfully picked berries—but never tried one. Mom made raspberry sauce for ice cream, put raspberries on oatmeal, served them plain and baked into muffins, but her son always said, "No, thank you." By week five she was working hard to not say, "You loved them when you were a baby! Please try one!" Then, with the last berries of the season on the table, he licked one, popped it in his mouth, and declared, "I like raspberries!"

The point isn't how many times or how many ways Mom offered berries. Waiting without comment—which felt nearly impossible at times—did the trick. This mom is convinced that had she tried to force her independent and anxious son to lick or try a tiny taste from day one, the endless negotiations would have spoiled the pleasure of picking them all summer, and he probably wouldn't have rediscovered that he liked raspberries. Some kids take baby steps and others wait and wait and then *just eat it* (as you may have been shouting in your head all along).

Ignore Initial Refusals

For most children (adventurous ones too) the first response *even to preferred foods* is "no," especially during the picky stage around fifteen months to four years, and will almost definitely be "no" for the child with EPE. Jenny's son went through a phase of yelling "No!" each time a food was offered. "Do you want chocolate cake?" (his favorite) was met with a loud "No!" then a pause and, "Wait, I mean yes!"

This right of first refusal gives children a much-needed sense of control. Not inviting immediate resistance is step one, and ignoring initial refusals is step two. Parents are amazed to learn this and watch their child happily eat a food that was adamantly refused minutes earlier. Ignoring initial refusals does not, of course, mean ignoring the child's wishes—it just means don't make it an issue. Try, for example: **"Say 'no thank you.' There are other things to eat."** Or **"Okay, you don't have to eat anything you don't want to."** Then move on.

What to Say and What Not to Say

If 95 percent of what you have been saying at meals was meant to convince your child to eat, you might not know what to talk about or how to talk about food without pressuring. Negotiating and therapy habits, such as "two more bites," will be hard to break. Essentially, your task is to ignore (or pretend to ignore) how much of what your child is or isn't eating. *You* set the mood at the table, so try staying calm and pleasant or at least neutral. The scripts throughout the book will guide you in ways to talk about food, but the best thing to talk about at mealtimes is anything *but* the food. Online resources for family meal topics and ideas are also easy to find. Here are a few examples to get you started:

"Who did you sit next to at lunch today?"

"What games did you play at recess?"

"If you could visit an island for a month, what three things would you take with you?"

"What's one good thing that happened today?"

Your child may feel put on the spot with direct questions. He may be happy to listen while you share with your partner or chat with a sibling. Try talking about yourself to get the dialogue going. Say: **"Guess what happened to me today!"** and then recount something your child can relate to. Or say: **"I saw Charlie's mom at the store. She told me she really enjoyed having you over last week."** Or: **"I was thinking we could go to the museum and see the new exhibit on mummies."**

Acknowledge Feelings, Then Say Yes and Soon

When your child isn't happy with the menu or the new routine, she may become upset. Acknowledge her emotions. Once you've done that to the best of your ability, the words "yes" and "soon" can prove invaluable. Sometimes a vague "yes" or "soon" is enough to satisfy your child (best for younger children). Say: **"It sounds like you're upset we aren't having pizza tonight. We'll have it again soon."** Or **"Yes, we'll have chicken nuggets again *soon*."** (Even if your child doesn't technically get what she wants, saying "yes" defuses conflict.) Sometimes your child may insist on pinning down "soon." In those cases, write it into the schedule. Say: **"We'll have yogurt again soon... When? Oh, let's write it in for snack tomorrow."**

Talking About New Foods

Particularly for children who like to know what to expect, briefly describing a new food helps them make a positive connection with past experiences and can increase acceptance. However, this is not a sales pitch, as in, "This is the best ever; it's so yummy; you'll love it;

it's sweet like candy!" Say: **"This is pasta like the macaroni, but the shape is different."** Or: **"It's not spicy."** Or: **"That's kohlrabi, I used to eat it as a kid in Germany. It tastes a little like broccoli stems."** Or: **"I cooked it the same way I cook carrots and peas."** Or: **"Oh, you like the teriyaki sauce on the noodles? The chicken has the same sauce."**

Find words with neutral or positive connotations for your child. One mom described how for a time she called every meat "chicken" ("chicken-pork" or "chicken-steak") to help her child understand the chewy characteristics of other meats. If your child pushes back, you could readjust, perhaps stepping back to more generic terms. For example, you might say, "This is like the vanilla yogurt you had yesterday." Your child responds, "No, it's totally different!" You readjust with, "This is vanilla."

Reframing "Encouragement" as "Facilitation"

"Encouragement" often turns into the "positive" pressure tactics described in chapter 3. One mom mused, "I was told to not pressure but *encourage* her, but I feel like everything I try turns into pressure." In the book *Promoting Positive Parenting*, authors Helen Woolley, Leezah Hertzmann, and Alan Stein describe "maternal facilitation," a great explanation of support without pressuring; it is "a measure of sensitive responsiveness, which refers to any maternal behavior that assists infants in an activity *in which they are engaged or seem ready to engage*" (2007, 112; emphasis ours).

The distinctions among "encouragement," "pressure," and "facilitation" are tricky, particularly if, in your family, encouragement ("try one bite") seems to help an easygoing sibling expand the variety of foods he eats. Facilitation might for example include holding out two spoons and letting the child choose, while pressure is spoon-feeding a child as he leans and twists away. Facilitation and support mean cutting apples into thin, peeled slices (more on food preparation in chapter 7), while pressure is holding a slice in front of his mouth and repeatedly asking, "Please try a bite."

While the authors refer to infants and moms, we believe all parents and children benefit from sensitive facilitation and response to the child's readiness and willingness to participate. (Hand a child a piece of food that she reaches for, help her hold and chew on her chew tube dipped in yogurt, and so on.) Bottom line? Regardless of the words used to describe it, you will know if what you are saying or doing has crossed into pressure by your child's reaction.

Talking About Food

Children with EPE are especially sensitive to food messaging, which they also hear on TV and at school. We introduce this topic because parents tell us they are scared to say the wrong things. Parents themselves may struggle with dieting or poor body image and find it difficult to talk about food in positive ways. Parents of girls, in particular, worry about feeding disorders morphing into eating disorders as they grow up in our thinness-obsessed culture (though boys develop eating disorders too).

Nutrition and Body Talk

Some think it's important to teach young children about nutrition or sustainability as a way to encourage eating "healthy" foods. We wonder why the rush, particularly when complex nutrition and health talk is hard for young children to grasp (Lytle et al. 1997). Nutrition talk can be especially problematic for children with EPE.

A child who is a competent eater may interpret messages such as "food = fuel" as interesting information (as in, candy gives quick energy, and oatmeal cookies or avocados give lasting energy and help you feel full because they contain fiber and fat). But say "Too much fat is bad for your heart," and the anxious child might frantically try to avoid all fat. When Jenny's son was four, a teacher pointed out the amount of sodium in a package of crackers and told the children to avoid foods with too much salt. Jenny's son demanded to know how much sodium was in everything he ate for the next six months, getting upset if it was "too high."

We live in a culture where children (and adults) find it almost impossible to feel good about food and their bodies. Increasingly, eating disorder and obesity-prevention experts stress that nutrition education focused on external cues (calorie counts, for example) rather than on self-regulation encourages disordered attitudes and eating (O'Dea and Wilson 2006; Neumark-Sztainer 2009). Pushing "healthy" foods can make children like them less (Maimaran and Fishbach 2014), while demonizing and forbidding "junk" foods can make many children obsess about, hide, and hoard these foods. A growing body of research tells us that how we think and feel about food impacts not only our enjoyment of food, but how we absorb nutrients and our ability to self-regulate as well! (There are dozens of studies, but our favorite is the 2011 "Mind over Milkshakes," by Crum and colleagues.)

In short, if nutrition talk helped your child be a healthier eater, you would have seen the results already. You will teach your child nutrition best by serving and enjoying a variety of foods.

> **Food for Thought:** Which of the following descriptions makes a food more appealing to you? Think about how you describe food to your child: healthy, high in protein, sweet, good for you, crunchy, salty, builds strong bones.

Here are a few ideas for talking about food in positive ways—though it's often best to say nothing, simply allowing your child to experience food for herself in a supportive atmosphere.

- Focus on joy and permission: **"We are lucky we get to eat so many wonderful foods: pizza and clementines, green beans and pie."** (The list of foods includes both "treats" and "healthy" foods.)

- Celebrate delicious food. Fruits and veggies taste good, too.

- Share other aspects of food, such as origin: **"We shop at the farmer's market because it's fun to meet the farmers who grow our food."**

- Respect body-size diversity: **"People come in all sizes, and that's just fine."**

- Be matter-of-fact about restrictions: **"Our family doesn't eat nuts because your brother could get really sick if he ate them, but we get to eat all kinds of other wonderful things."**

- Create and celebrate food traditions with your children.

- Be age-appropriate; young children can learn that a banana is a fruit, but may not understand "protein."

Try to avoid messages that judge, such as "Candy (sugar, flour, meat) is bad" or "That's junk." Children as young as four report feeling guilt and shame when eating forbidden foods (Fisher and Birch 2000). Young children tend to think that if a food is "bad," and they enjoy it, then *they* are bad too. Try not to let your children hear you say, "I was so bad, I (had dessert, ate too much)" or "I was good, I didn't (eat dessert, eat too much)." Avoid praising or judging children around eating ("Olivia is a good, healthy eater, but Ethan is our picky sugar addict") or inciting shame or fear ("If you don't [eat X or avoid Y] you will get sick and fat"). Even kinder, gentler labels can backfire, including "green-light" or "red-light" foods; "growing" or "fun" foods; or "healthy" and "unhealthy" foods. Children can still hear "good" and "bad."

Talking About Treats

You've probably noticed that, in STEPS+, unlike other foods served at meals, dessert is limited (more on treats in the next chapter). Your child will notice too! How can you explain this?

We've found that the generic word "treat," when used to describe sweets, pricier foods like avocados or organic meats, eating out, the ripest fruits, or foods that take a lot of time or effort to cook, keeps all food on a level playing field. You might say: **"What a treat to get ice cream on such a hot day after your game!"** Or **"This steak is such a treat."** Or **"What a treat that Grandma cooked lasagna for us!"** And even **"Spending the whole afternoon with you is such a treat!"** When older kids ask, "Why can't I eat more ice cream? You let me eat all the crackers I want," you might answer: **"We get to eat all kinds of foods: ice cream, crackers, apples, peas. If we eat only ice cream, we wouldn't feel good; if we eat only broccoli, that wouldn't be balanced either."**

Messages That Respect Everyone's Needs

Siblings can feel ignored or slighted with the attention focused on the child with EPE. Or you may be dealing with EPE in one child, a preoccupation with sweets in another, and a concern about rapid weight gain in another (or maybe even in your child with EPE). The approach in this book applies to all your children, instilling positive attitudes and behaviors around food and weight. With a smaller than average child, obesity may be the last thing on your mind, but most adults who struggle with weight were in the normal or underweight range as children. Teaching your children (big or small) to eat based on internal hunger cues should help them achieve a stable and healthy weight as well as improved health life-long (Van Dyke and Drinkwater 2013). And by feeding all your children the same way, you aren't comparing or implying that one child is better because of what she eats or how she looks, and you won't send mixed messages.

We have many client families where one parent is picky, or avoids gluten because doing so feels better. In such a case, you might say: **"Daddy's tummy doesn't feel good if he eats those noodles, but he has other things he likes to eat."** In general, if adults set the tone and don't make a big deal about not being able (or wanting) to eat X,

Y, or Z, or comment about how "gross" A, B, or C is, children can grow up feeling good about food. If one parent follows a restrictive plan (like paleo or Atkins), is dieting, or is weighing portions or counting points, he or she can hopefully do so discreetly and without comment so as not to confuse the children.

Eating Away from Home

You probably won't be able to (or want to) eat every meal or snack together at home, and depending upon work and school schedules, you may eat separately as often as you eat together. This section covers eating together in restaurants or at friends' houses, and your child's experience when visiting another's home or spending time with a nanny or daycare provider.

Family Meals in Restaurants

Whether you eat out once a month or three times a week, you can enjoy meals together away from home—where your child may even be more willing to try new foods. In the beginning, make the goal about reducing anxiety. Later in the process, you can think more about balanced options (see chapter 7).

Here are some suggestions for adapting the family meal to dining out:

- Start with family-friendly restaurants.

- Try to go when it's not busy so you won't have long to wait.

- Bring a small container of dry cereal or crackers (a "tide-me-over") in case there is a longer-than-expected wait with a hungry and impatient child.

- To deal with wait time, stock a small bag with activities like puzzle books, crayons, and stickers, and keep it by the door so you can grab it and go. A handheld game or smartphone may make the wait bearable until your child is more comfortable at the table. Put the games away when the food arrives.

- Buffets provide a relatively cost-effective way to expose your child to new tastes. Fill a plate or two with small amounts of different foods ("appetizers") and put them in the middle of the table. Offer a few sauces for dips.

- Indian, Thai, or Chinese buffets often have white rice or naan bread that are accepted by many children with EPE.

- A booth provides peace of mind (no tipping chairs) and gives your child stability. If it helps him settle, allow him to take off his shoes and sit cross-legged.

- Order a side or two of accepted foods like bread or pasta. Many restaurants happily accommodate; no need to explain. Say: **"May we have a side of plain pasta, with sauce on the side?"** Or: **"Can we have an extra plate so we can share?"** Or: **"Could you please bring a small scoop of vanilla ice cream with the rest of the meal?"** Or: **"Would you please bring more of your white bread? I'm happy to pay for extra."**

- Rotate through two or three restaurants at which you have had success. Familiar places may encourage curiosity.

- If there is no buffet, help your child order. With young children, you might order a side she generally likes or share your entree. Siblings can also share an entree.

Most restaurants have at least one thing most children with EPE can eat: bread, plain pasta, fries, corn, or ice cream. If your child enjoys the meal, maybe only eating fries or ice cream, that's okay for now. A tear-free meal with smiles is progress. And if he doesn't eat what he ordered, don't make it a big deal (just like at home); maybe take it for your own lunch the next day. One mom anticipated that her son wouldn't eat what he ordered, but was happy he was comfortable ordering something new.

If your child hasn't had success finding something he can eat in restaurants, consider reviewing menu options online together. Say: **"We're trying a new restaurant tonight. Let's take a look at the menu and see what might look good. Ooh, I might try the chicken and pasta!"** (Choosing while your server waits pen-in-hand or with others commenting might be enough stress to shut down appetite.) If you are heading to a familiar restaurant, discuss two or three items he has enjoyed before. Choosing in advance can reduce anxiety at the restaurant, but give him the option to change his mind before it's time to order.

Sometimes, especially if you are traveling, you have little control over where to eat. If there are no good options for your child, then bringing a safe food is reasonable. Doing so discreetly will keep your child from feeling like the focus: perhaps bring a baggie of accepted crackers that he can put on his bread plate. Ideally, this will be transitional and he can gradually move to ordering off the menu, even if it's a side of plain pasta.

Some children may always need foods from home if they are tube-fed or have severe oral motor problems, and our society should accommodate that. Unfortunately, you may have to protect your child from comments from other diners and even waitstaff. Most wouldn't think to comment, but some staff and even text on children's menus interfere with children and eating (by saying, for example, "If you eat all your meal, you can ask your parents if you can have a cookie"). See chapter 4 for responses to others who pressure your child to eat.

Sometimes, in spite of trying all the strategies above, eating out can be such a source of anxiety that you might choose to eat in as much as you can while getting your other steps in place. (Ideas for cooking and what to serve at home are in chapter 7.) You can transition to eating away from home with baby steps: getting take-out from a restaurant before eating there, starting with an ice-cream parlor, or eating at a best friend's house.

Eating at Friends' Houses

When you are invited to a neighbor's house for dinner, you may feel embarrassed by your child's eating or find that it becomes a topic of conversation. Remember that you decide how much to tell and to whom. No one "deserves" or needs details. A good strategy is to acknowledge a comment without apologizing or explaining, then change the subject: **"Yep, we all have our issues, don't we? Hey, how was the school fundraiser?"** Or **"Oh? I'm not concerned that she only ate bread for dinner. Can you please pass the chicken?"**

Some parents use social gatherings as leverage to get children to eat: "If you won't eat anything they have, we aren't going for dinner!" Avoid this. Your child already feels singled out for her eating and the threat is unlikely to motivate her to eat. Threats and shame are likely to make her more self-conscious, make her a target for siblings ("We aren't going because of you!"), and increase her anxiety (decreasing appetite). Bring a safe food to share, plan a bedtime snack when you get home, and enjoy your friends' company.

Exercise: List foods your child eats that you could bring to share. Chips and salsa? (Even if he only eats the chips.) Bread and spinach dip? (Even if he only eats the bread.) Veggie tray? (Even if he only eats cucumbers.)

The goal, for you and your child, is to have a good time with friends. Occasionally, when children are having fun at parties or at school and their peers are eating, they may branch out. One mom of a child with EPE explained how Jessie came home from preschool talking about "Max's cheese." At the store, they found slices like Max's (Colby-Jack), and Jessie pulled one into small pieces and ate it, to her mother's astonishment! Jessie saw the cheese in a different context, free from past negative associations.

Eating with Babysitters or at Day Care

It's likely that your child sometimes (or often) eats at day care or with a childcare provider (we will use "she" for the sake of simplicity) either in your home, in the provider's home, or at a center. As the parent of a child with EPE, you may have already had difficult conversations about your child's eating with his care providers. Any time we question how childcare providers feed or ask them to change, they may feel judged, or even that their jobs are at stake. Nannies who have cared for many children spanning a number of years may react negatively if how they feed children is a source of pride. It can be even trickier if grandparents or family members provide child care ("I fed you this way and you turned out fine!").

Altogether, it can feel like a sensitive subject. But it's important to make the effort to get your childcare provider on board with the changes you are making around feeding.

It helps to remember that babysitters and childcare providers genuinely care for children and want the best for them. Looking at feeding issues from your childcare provider's perspective helps. First, she'll have her own style. Your childcare provider was once a child, raised with her family's own food rules. She may also have raised (or be raising) her own children a certain way with food—like the rest of America, probably not the way we advocate in this book. She may use an authoritarian approach ("You will sit until you eat it all") or be more permissive ("You want some candy? Okay. You can eat later if you want.")

Many providers are asked by some parents to push food on their children, or restrict it. Childcare providers may feel like it is their job to improve children's nutrition and vegetable intake, especially if the first thing parents do at pick-up is ask for detailed information about what and how much a child ate.

Here are some tips that may help you have a constructive conversation about feeding with your child's care provider:

- If one parent is less emotional about the topic, have that person lead the discussion.

138

- Start by thanking her for her efforts and acknowledging that you know that, like you, she wants the best for the child.

- Tell her that you are trying a new way of feeding if you have been asking her to push intake. Be specific so she doesn't have to guess what you want. It may help to share the "Essentials" handout (in our online resources at http://www.newharbinger.com/31106) with her.

- Once you have your mealtime routine down, ask your nanny to stay for dinner a few times so you can model how you would like meals to go.

When you establish a respectful and thoughtful dialogue with your nanny about feeding, you'll benefit from her thoughts and observations about mealtimes with your child. You might find that she just needs permission to stop pressuring, and will embrace the changes you are asking her to make.

Regulated childcare centers may have specific food rules, especially if they participate in government programs. This can mean that food is preplated or that the child can't have seconds of a preferred food before eating other items. A doctor's note can help with special requests in these situations. Or you may need to make a change in childcare center if the tension and confusion of mixed messages are making eating harder for your child.

We hope these ideas get your family on track to enjoyable meals together. Work on establishing routine and connecting at the table before diverting too much energy to menu planning—the subject of the next chapter, chapter 7. In addition, if your child has significant oral-motor or sensory challenges, consider skipping to chapter 8 and coming back to chapter 7. If you feel ready, or if not having ideas for what to put on the table is a major hurdle, then read on for guidance on what to serve, and how.

Step 4: Know What to Serve and How to Serve It

How you feed is more important right now than *what*, and a happy mood at the table will make everyone's food taste better. As Aesop wrote, "A crust eaten in peace is better than a banquet partaken in anxiety." However, parents often find that figuring out what to serve feels paralyzing, and that ideas for foods and different preparations can help them think more creatively—and make it to the table! In this chapter, you will learn techniques for food planning, preparation, and presentation, with a bit of menu inspiration thrown in. Whatever your level of comfort in the kitchen, if your attitude conveys warmth and calm, it will go a long way toward making both kitchen and table a place where your child wants to be.

Menu Plan for the Whole Family

Too often, a family's menu is limited by the preferences of the child with EPE. Many parents mourn the loss of their own favorites, and those who used to enjoy cooking may feel defeated. But you can get out of that kid-food rut!

"What do *I* want to eat?" This simple question gets lost in the shuffle of trying to meet everyone else's needs, but if you are the primary cook and menu planner, you decide what's on the menu. Having a child with EPE can feel like you are using a cookbook with 98 percent of the pages missing. Bringing back your favorite dishes gives *you* something to look forward to. When you sit down to foods you actually want to eat, not only do you expose your child to a wider variety of foods, but you can also authentically model enjoying different foods.

Exercise: List foods you like and used to cook, or want to learn to make: main dishes, soups, stews, sides, fruits, desserts. Pull out your family recipe book or favorite cookbooks for inspiration.

But don't let your preferences limit the menu if you aren't an adventurous eater. Your child is his own person, and will have unique preferences, which might not match yours. Don't be afraid to offer "adult" flavors: Katja remembers dining with friends whose toddler ignored the soft bread and gobbled up pickled ginger. Many children with sensory issues prefer strong salty, savory, sour, tart, or spicy flavors, eating wasabi peas, lemon slices, or hot salsa by the spoonful. Particularly for sensory seekers, offering intense flavors, even ones you wouldn't consider, can broaden her accepted foods.

Just Say No to Short-Order Cooking

Trying to satisfy each family member's likes and dislikes at every meal is overwhelming, and there is a better way. By rotating variety, you will hit on each family member's favorites at least every few days. Safe foods that satisfy your child with EPE (that everyone can enjoy) may appear more often than other foods, and that's okay.

Exercise: Make a list of foods your child eats or has eaten: In one column, list his almost-always accepted or *safe* foods. In a separate column, list foods he *sometimes* eats. Then list foods he *has eaten* in the past. Observe or ask if your child prefers salty, sweet, crunchy, or smooth tastes and textures. List all accepted condiments.

Make a list of foods you know how to make or *want* to eat on the back of or next to your child's lists. Consider consolidating into one format with main dishes, sides, and so on.

Once you have the lists suggested in the above exercise, circle any options the whole family can enjoy that you can serve more often. Keep the lists on the side of the fridge or in a drawer where you, the parent, can see them. Add or move foods as your child's preferences change. Here is what the lists for your child with EPE might look like:

Safe foods: crackers (Ritz, club), pretzels, plain pasta, rice, French toast fingers, McDonalds plain hamburger, chicken nuggets, vanilla tube yogurt, maple instant oatmeal

Sometimes-eats foods: canned mandarin oranges, seedless red grapes cut in half, vanilla yogurt from a cup, Wheat Thins, plain peas

Has eaten: frozen peas, baked potato, shredded cheese, plain meatballs, cherry-flavored Popsicle, sugar cookie, oatmeal made with water

Has refused: fresh fruit or vegetables, mixed textures, most meats

Prefers: sweet, salty, and smooth

Condiments: ketchup and ranch dressing

When planning dinner, lunch, or snack, serve foods *you* want to eat, or foods you want your children to learn to like. Initially, include one or two foods from the safe foods list. It might feel silly to serve store-bought rotisserie chicken with microwaved frozen peas and mashed potatoes next to a bowl of pretzels, but if your child comes to the table and sees *something* she can eat, and knows she won't be pressured to eat other foods, she can relax, look around, smell, pass, maybe poke, and eventually try new foods.

143

Here is a sample menu that combines the preferences and safe foods of a child with EPE and her parent:

Breakfast: French toast fingers, yogurt from a cup, and cut-up bananas (the child cuts the bananas if she is willing and able). The parent is also eating scrambled eggs; she makes a bit extra, puts them on a serving plate, and serves herself.

Morning snack: Pretzels, canned mandarin oranges, and tube yogurt (whole-fat milk, as the child likes it and increasing fat is a goal).

Lunch: Whole-grain crackers, pita bread quarters, whipped cream cheese with a spreader so the child can apply it, turkey lunchmeat, and grapes. Since she is old enough, the child eats the grapes whole or cuts them herself with an appropriate knife. The parent wants pita bread and turkey with avocado, so she slices some avocado and puts it on a plate on the table so the child sees it and can help herself.

Snack: Cut-up apple with half the slices peeled, cinnamon-sugar shaker on the table, chicken nuggets, and pretzels.

Dinner: Plain rice, rotisserie chicken, microwaved peas, panfried onion and peppers with teriyaki sauce (the parent uses presliced vegetables), ketchup on the table, and vanilla frozen yogurt for dessert.

How long you serve favored foods, and for how many meals and snacks a day, will vary. If your child has few safe foods, have something from his favored list *at every meal or snack* while you get the hang of keeping a routine and avoiding pressure. Once you have been doing this for a while or his anxiety has improved, try one meal or snack per day where you offer only from the "sometimes eats" list, knowing that in a few hours he will have the chance to eat a favored food again.

Family menus limited to the preferences of the most selective child make it harder for siblings to eat well. Parents often share that a major motivation to tackle meal planning is a younger sibling dropping certain foods and emulating the negotiating and poor mealtime behaviors of the child with EPE. One dad said: "Our younger son now loves lentils. I don't think he'd ever had them. We are more aware of not limiting his opportunities."

Supporting Nutrition Within the Menu

While parents are working on the steps and meal-planning, many children with EPE can meet their basic nutrition needs; others with more limited intake benefit from nutrition support. In addition to any accepted multivitamin or DHA chew, there are ways to support nutrition without pressure. Consider nutritionally dense and varied forms of accepted foods. For example, substitute whole grains for refined grains: offer whole-grain versions of crackers, white bread, or toaster waffles.

What About Supplements?

One of the first "solutions" your doctor may have recommended is a nutrition supplement drink or flavored cereal or protein bar offered continuously throughout the day. With the sweet and easy supplement drink as an option, appetite is sabotaged and many children with EPE increasingly rely on the supplements, eating less and less—to their parents' frustration. This is especially likely if there has been pressure around eating or if there are unaddressed oral motor problems. Here are tips to include supplements that don't undermine your child's appetite or progress:

- If supplement drinks are your child's primary source of nutrition or you are scared to stop offering them, start by serving them with meals and snacks (not between).

- Rotate brands and flavors so your child doesn't get stuck on one.

- Serve from cups or neutral bowls or plates so your child doesn't fixate on packaging.

- Powdered mixes, such as Carnation Instant Breakfast or Ovaltine, are cheaper than premixed drinks like PediaSure. Start with a small amount of powder in milk or an accepted beverage and increase as your child gets used to it.

- Make smoothies mixed with ingredients like cow's milk, soy or almond milk, yogurt, vegetables, fruits, protein powders, or nut butters. Ask your dietitian for recommendations. Ingredients you might not consider could be just what your child likes: instant breakfast mix, baby rice cereal, peanut butter, bananas, mangoes.

Sneak with Caution

Due to the popularity of "sneaking" cookbooks, many parents try hiding nutrient-dense foods like yams in mac 'n' cheese. We've heard of moms baking brownies furtively at night, taking spinach containers to the garage trash to hide the evidence. But sneaking can backfire. Moms who sneak suspect, correctly, that if they are discovered, their children will become distrustful. And for the child with EPE, it's hard to sneak anything into plain noodles, so sneaking isn't the answer. If sneaking is working for you, proceed with caution. But if you don't want your child to know you're sneaking, you may want to reconsider your approach. Chances are, he might not care either way, so if you do add foods or purees to support nutrition, do so in the open so that you aren't "sneaking." You are simply preparing food. Here are some ways to do it:

- Add shredded or blended carrots or zucchini (start with peeled) to muffins. Let your child push the button on the food processor.

- Add pureed carrots or sweet potatoes to spaghetti sauce.

- Make pancakes with sweet potatoes. Have your child help you make the batter, so she sees what is going in.

- Try one-quarter whole-wheat pastry flour and three-quarters all-purpose flour in place of all-purpose flour in recipes.

- Add applesauce to baked goods.

Initially you might want to serve the new version with the old favorite, or the new pancakes with accepted sides. It might be best to let your child know in advance so he doesn't also reject the "safe" version, wondering if it has been tinkered with. Say: **"I tried using different ingredients with half the pancakes this time."**

Juicing or Pureeing

Some clients have had good luck with juicers. Many children enjoy putting the foods in and watching the juice dribble out. Even if you strain the juice, as many parents do initially for it to be accepted, it still introduces flavors and boosts nutrition. If you can afford it, a Vitamix blender blends so powerfully that most of the texture disappears. Vitamix smoothies or frozen pops with fruits—or even spinach—may be accepted, while the same preparations would be rejected from a standard food processor or blender that leaves traces of apple skin or spinach stalk. (Some insurers cover Vitamix blenders for homemade tube feeds.)

If you use supplements, mix nutrient-dense foods into baked goods, or use shakes, juices, and frozen pops to support nutrition, be sure to expose your children to the foods in their whole forms. Let's take blueberries:

- Bake them into muffins, or buy a blueberry muffin if you don't bake.

- Make half a batch of pancakes with blueberries.

- Offer frozen blueberries in a bowl if your child has adequate oral motor skills. Your child might especially like frozen fruits or veggies.

- Serve freeze-dried blueberries to a child who likes crunch, or dried or yogurt-covered blueberries to a child who prefers chewy.

- Serve blueberries in yogurt or buy blueberry-flavored yogurt of a brand your child already likes.

- Try blueberry jam.

- Make yogurt, ice cream, or oatmeal "sundaes" with different bowls of toppings, including blueberries.

Sometimes even with all these nutrition-boosting ideas, your child may still not get what he needs by mouth. Work with a registered pediatric dietitian, follow your child's growth, and find support. Before resorting to restraining or force-feeding your child, consider supplementing intake through tube-feeding. Refer to chapter 4 for considerations about tube feeds.

When You Don't or Can't Cook

If you aren't serving foods because you don't enjoy cooking, don't know how, or don't have the time, prepared foods can help. Getting food to the table is the priority, and any assistance is worth exploring. You can learn about cooking when you have the time and energy (when you're ready, try a cooking class with a friend or make it a "girls'" or "'boys' night out" where you have fun, learn something new, and get inspired).

Options to help get meals on the table with little or no cooking include:

- Microwaveable bags of vegetables and entrees

- Take-and-bake bread (or pizza)

- Fresh pasta, requiring a quick boil, served with premade sauce

- Prewashed salads, prechopped veggies, and precut fruits

- Prepared frozen meals you put in the slow cooker in the morning

- Packaged sausage fully cooked and ready to heat in the microwave or on the stovetop

- Rotisserie chicken whole or from the deli section with the meat already off the bones

- Meal prep centers, where you go to make batches of freezer meals; find them online at the Easy Meal Prep Association website

- Let others cook for you: Ask for gift certificates or cooking services as birthday or anniversary gifts, and if friends offer to help in a crisis, ask them to drop off a meal.

- In addition to friends and family, stores that have readymade family meals you can pick up on your way home, or meal prep services that deliver to your workplace

- Many chain restaurants are adding menu options that support eating family style, like entrees or orders of side dishes that serve four.

One appliance that streamlines home cooking is a second freezer. If you have the space and resources, having one can make shopping with a time and money budget easier: you can freeze meals in batches, freeze meats on sale, and buy in quantity and freeze breads or fruits for smoothies. Specialty drinks or foods for allergies can be pricey, so finding them on sale or buying in bulk and freezing saves money.

Getting Organized

Half the task of planning and getting meals on the table is organization. It takes time and trial and error! There will be nights when the only thing between your family and dinner is a missing can of tomato

149

sauce. Plan ahead as much as you can. Start with a rough menu for a weekend of meals and snacks, filled with the foods you eat now. If you order pizza, write that into the plan.

Plan a trip to the grocery store to stock your pantry and fridge with easy-to-prepare and quick-grab items for snacks or meals away from home—baby carrots, yogurt tubes, string cheese, cereal bars, milk boxes, raisins, dehydrated fruit, applesauce pouches, crackers, and so on. Try a mix of foods your child is comfortable with and foods that he is working on, and always have something safe available.

Find a general resource for new cooks—like Ellyn Satter's *Secrets of Feeding a Healthy Family* (2011)—with recipes, advice for stocking a pantry, and sample menus. *The America's Test Kitchen Quick Family Cookbook* is another good source for everything from essential gear to last-minute sides. Apps, websites, or free cookbook software help you plan and stay organized: try Spinning Meals, AllRecipe, Epicurious, Yummly, BigOven, Tony's Recipe Cookbook, or plantoeat.com, among others.

Block off a weekend to clear out your cupboards or pantry and start fresh. Send the kids to Grandma's or ask a friend to help. Toss expired foods, and donate items you don't want to cook or eat. Organize canned goods, pastas, spices, and so on. Make a list of pantry basics you're missing, using one of the resources listed above for inspiration if you like. If you are really stuck, there are people you can hire to organize your kitchen and pantry!

Consider Your Child's Skills and Preferences

If your child with EPE is struggling with specific oral motor skills or textures, find foods that match her skills and tolerance. Children tend toward the path of least resistance (don't we all?), but making things comfortable isn't about only serving foods that are already safe. Pulling together what you know about your child's skills and the characteristics of various foods and using a little creativity will go a long way toward expanding what might be accepted. Here is a reference list of types of foods and the oral motor skills required, for when you need ideas for foods your child can handle and next-step foods to challenge and improve her skills.

Purees

Foods include stage 1 and 2 baby food, applesauce, yogurt, pudding, blended meals, blended pasta, and meats blended with broth

Oral motor skills needed include sucking (tongue moves up and down) or suckling (tongue moves in and out), and the ability to close lips around spoon and food

Lumpy Purees

Foods include guacamole, refried beans, fork-mashed banana, fork-mashed ravioli in sauce, oatmeal, hummus, finely ground or blended chicken salad, and yogurt with soft fruit pieces

Oral motor skills needed include sucking or suckling, the ability to close lips around spoon and food, and up-and-down jaw and tongue movement

Ground or Soft Solid Texture

Foods include hamburger, ground turkey or chicken, chicken nuggets, fish sticks, sloppy joes, roasted potato without skin, avocado, banana chunks, soft pasta (ravioli, bowtie, tortellini), soft breads, fish, French fries, rice, and beans

Oral motor skills needed include sucking or suckling, the ability to close lips around spoon and food, and up-and-down jaw and tongue movement with simple side-to-side tongue movement

Coarsely Chopped

Foods include fruit cocktail, diced steamed veggies, diced raw soft vegetables (cucumber, tomatoes) or fruits (kiwi, peaches, strawberries), crackers, chips, baked chicken, and softer nuts such as cashews

Oral motor skills include sucking or suckling, the ability to close lips around spoon and food, up-and-down jaw and tongue movement, side-to-side tongue movement, and vertical and diagonal jaw movement, with strength to break up the pieces

Dual, Multiple, or Difficult Textures

Foods include unpeeled apple, grapes, blueberries, orange segments, sandwiches, vegetable soup, steak, hard raw vegetables (carrots, celery, peppers), and hard nuts such as almonds

Oral motor skills include sucking or suckling, closing lips around spoon and food, up-and-down jaw and tongue movement, side-to-side tongue movement, vertical, diagonal, and rotary jaw movement, with strength to grind up pieces, and controlled, sustained bite on something hard at the molars

Many children progress from thin to thicker purees as described above; however, children with oral motor problems may not tolerate runny foods that move quickly in the mouth. It seems counterintuitive, but these children often do best with *thicker* consistencies such as purees with added baby rice or oatmeal cereal.

Sensory Preference Matching

For the sensory seeker, try crunchy alternatives or additions to foods you've tried. Having a crunchy item on the table that your child can alternate with other foods may help him maintain oral awareness. Vegetables and fruits come in a wide assortment of crunchy and chewy varieties, ranging from freeze-dried to dried and roasted and from salty to sweet. Many children need a specific combination of crunchy but meltable—think Garden Veggie Straws or Gerber Graduates Puffs, which dissolve with little chewing. Cheerios, a common first crunchy food given to infants, aren't as dissolvable.

Many sensory seekers crave strong flavors; Jenny says that Cheetos Puffs are a preferred starter food for her clients for this very reason!

Exercise: If your child can only munch up and down or with his front teeth, do that yourself and see what happens. Trying food before you give it to your child helps you better understand if and how he may struggle.

Think Outside the Box (or Recipe)

There are thousands of cookbooks, and no end of recipes on the Internet. Considering your child's preferences, search specifically for different (for you!) ways of preparing familiar foods. When Jenny's son gave up broccoli after eating it as a toddler, she tried something different. He loved soy sauce, so she served broccoli with soy sauce for dipping and voilà—he ate it up! Children who love crunchy or salty foods may like veggies oven-roasted with Parmesan sprinkled on top and baked crispy, or a roasted vegetable with coarse sea salt.

Many successful home cooks build a repertoire of meals that show up regularly. Katja has found that for every four new recipes she tries, one might make the cut, with considerations for complexity, cost, and taste. Let your family join the process of rating new recipes. Who liked what and why? A delicious stew that takes three hours to make won't show up often if there is a tasty and less complicated alternative. If you know a great family cook, ask questions, watch her cook, ask for recipes, and nose around in her pantry (with permission!).

Introducing New Foods

Check out your supermarket for new vegetables and fruits or head to the farmer's market. If you are concerned that what you buy won't get eaten, wasting food and money, buy one Asian pear or zucchini, or a snack pack of a new cracker rather than an entire box. Know that wasting food is part of the process—for a while. Redefine waste—if you don't offer new or challenging foods, that's a wasted *opportunity*! A child with permission not to eat is more likely to try something new. To minimize waste:

- Buy small amounts or share with another family.

- Make smaller portions of new foods.

- Serve foods in bowls with lids and put leftovers directly in the fridge.

- Cook and freeze.

- Look for sales on unfamiliar items.

Try a weekly family "tasting" night to explore a new recipe or food without pressure. If you find a winner, buy more next time. Jenny's oldest son discovered jicama after his Spanish teacher mentioned it. He thought the name was awesome and asked Jenny to buy some. She had never tried it herself, but they read about it online and tried crunchy jicama slices with almond butter for snack: it became a new family favorite!

Preparing and Serving Meats

Worry about protein intake, or children not eating meat, is a major concern for many parents dealing with extreme picky eating. Chicken nuggets are often the only meat their child eats. It's understandable when you consider that the crunchy (but not thick) breading is just right for a child who needs more input, while the chicken requires little chewing. Chicken nuggets show up often on the safe foods list for children Jenny diagnoses with chewing problems.

Many meats are tough or chewy. The child with poor jaw and tongue stability or coordination chews and chews—and then spits it out. The child with texture hypersensitivity might put it in his mouth—then spit it out. It doesn't take long to figure out which meats he can handle and which to postpone. Preparing meats in enticing ways that match your child's skill level optimizes your chances of success. Here are some tips:

- Remember to provide a paper napkin so he has a discreet option for spitting out food.

- Use a slow cooker to soften meats and break down some of the tougher fibers.

- Mix new with familiar foods. Try chicken nuggets with whole-grain breading, or make your own at home. Serve the new version beside the tried and true on one plate so that they are presented the same way. Allow him to choose the ones he recognizes without comment.

- Use the broiler to crisp the outside of meats, or panfry to get a crispy coating on breaded chicken, tofu, or even scrambled eggs. Get Shake 'n Bake bags or make your own crunchy coating with an accepted cracker, like Ritz or Goldfish. Fry bacon to extra crispy, or microwave pepperoni to make it crunchy.

- Use favored condiments (tomato sauce, ranch dressing, ketchup, teriyaki, soy sauce) to coat chicken, turkey, or beef (including meatballs or ground meat crumbles) when cooking, or as a dipping sauce. Serve ground meats with accepted sauces, like sloppy joes, mild (or hot) taco or chili seasoning, or meat sauce with spaghetti.

- Change how it looks. Cut deli meats or cheeses into shapes with cookie cutters, make kabobs with pieces of chicken, or prepare small squares of chicken, deli meat, or shrimp. When served with cheese, crackers, and a spread (hummus, guacamole, cream cheese), your child can put together fancy hors d'oeuvres.

- Offer meats without breading like roasted chicken or tender pork cuts if your child has the oral motor skills. Even if she chews the meat and spits it out, she gets the flavor and some iron, and is working on chewing.

- Make the size more manageable. A whole hamburger patty may overwhelm, but a patty cut into "meatballs" may feel more doable; or make sliders with smaller buns.

- Try mini hot dogs or corn dogs.

- Shred chicken in a food processor and serve it in a bowl to put on crackers or eat with a spoon. Add sauces, dips, or broth to moisten.

Preparing and Serving Fruits and Veggies

Poor intake of vegetables, and fruits to a lesser extent, is often high on the list of parents' worries. Vegetables don't always lend themselves to a child's preferences—they are, quite honestly, harder to learn to like. Fruits are sweeter and easier to like, but the wet quality and seeds of some fruits can be a turn-off. Try new presentations or condiments to increase opportunities to explore. For example:

- Serve raw versions of veggies you cook with a meal, or with the "tide-me-over."

- Include dips (hummus, peanut butter, caramel, yogurt, sour cream and onion), ranch or yogurt dressings, ketchup, or other condiments.

- Keep serving veggies, without comment—don't forget snacks.

- Serve veggies different ways. Your child might reject a baby carrot but might eat coin-shaped carrot pieces, roasted carrot chips, or matchstick carrots.

- Add fat, flavor, and even sugar. Adding a little sugar helps many children overcome the bitter taste of some vegetables.

Simmer chopped carrots in broth and half a teaspoon of brown sugar or honey and a little butter.

- Try roasted vegetables: sweet potato, squash, carrot, green beans, taro, and even okra. They are crunchy and a bit salty—a flavor and texture that might resemble those of your child's favorite potato chip.

- Bulk bins offer options: dried mangoes, yogurt-covered raisins, dates, veggie chips—buy a little to try.

- Put out different toppings (sesame seeds, crunchy wonton noodles) with a meal and include salad or vegetables.

Looks Matter

Your child with EPE might be put off by visual chaos: foods that touch each other or look different. The shape, size, and look of food changes every time she takes a bite, and this can create anxiety in a child who dislikes change. Most children go through a phase where they turn up their noses at foods with visible spices or vegetables. If your child needs to pick out berries from a muffin or eat around the edges of a casserole, let him, without comment. Let him cut crusts off breads, or do it for him.

Many children pick up on changes in the appearance of a food or even a serving container. Avoid serving foods from the original containers when possible. Your child may latch onto the familiar label, creating an impossible situation if the manufacturer decides to change it or you can't get that specific container. Here are some tips:

- Bring a bowl to the table with the preferred container and show your child how he can spoon food into his bowl. He sees that moving it from one container to another doesn't change it.

- Leave out spices, pepper, or chopped herbs while cooking and let everyone add their own at the table.

- Place serving bowls at an accepted distance from your child and allow him to have his own multiple small bowls or a cafeteria-style tray.

- Ask your child if he wants something cut up or not—it is easier to cut something than to put it back together, and he may want to pick it up and bite off pieces.

Hot or Cold

Consider how temperature changes the consistency and appeal of foods, like oatmeal. Would you eat warm shrimp cocktail or cold beef stew? Your child has her own preferences. If your child prefers foods at room temperature, add ice cubes to hot soups or stews, place the food in the fridge briefly to cool off, stir the food, or teach her to blow on it to cool it off. If a food has cooled and your child prefers it hot, you (or your older child) can microwave it during the meal. For the child who prefers cold foods, try frozen fruits and veggies, yogurt, or smoothie pops to introduce flavors, or serve foods straight from the refrigerator.

Building Bridges to New Foods

Learning to like new foods is something like learning a new language. If you are immersed in a language, you learn because you have to communicate your needs and wants, and it happens in a natural way. *Food immersion* happens when your child sits at the table with you every day—becoming fluent in the foods your family eats. But your child will need bridges he can cross to access your family foods. Building those bridges can make all the difference.

Realistic Expectations

You wouldn't expect a child with motor delays to learn to ride a bicycle at the same age as his typically developing peers, or in one afternoon. When parents have unrealistic expectations for how long it will take for a child to eat a more typical variety of foods, it's hard for them to see the progress that is happening. Even when your child sees foods over and over, it takes time. A sibling might branch out after two or ten exposures, but the child with EPE may need dozens or hundreds. Don't get discouraged and give up before your child has a chance to make those first tentative steps toward the bridge.

When There Is No Bridge

If your child is only eating processed, high-flavor, or fast foods, and you only eat plain, low-fat foods such as broiled chicken or fish and steamed veggies, expecting him to make the leap to your relatively bland foods will be an obstacle. As one dad put it, "I just don't see how he can go from eating nuggets and waffles to quinoa and broiled chicken." Frankly, neither can we. If you eat foods solely for their perceived health benefits and taste isn't important, your child has little motivation to branch out. There is no bridge over that gaping canyon.

Children, particularly those who struggle with eating, aren't motivated to eat for health benefits they can't comprehend. If you yourself eat for fuel or for health, it may feel difficult or like an imposition to change the foods you serve. But your child will make progress only if she enjoys what she tries, and most people prefer foods with some fat and flavor.

Bridging by Chaining or Fading

You can help your child transition to new foods via characteristics (flavor and texture) of foods she already enjoys. This idea has been called linking or bridging, but is most often referred to as "food chaining," a term coined by Cheri Fraker (Fraker et al. 2009). The book by the same name includes, among other helpful suggestions, lists of foods to move along, or chain. For instance, if your child likes cheese, you might cross over to a cheese-flavored cracker, put cheese sauce on broccoli, or mix cheese into scrambled eggs. If he likes crunchy and sweet, try kettle popcorn, or dehydrated pineapple slices. Even condiments can provide that bridge.

Exercise: Name two or three characteristics for each food on the list of your child's safe foods. Is it crunchy or smooth? Savory or sweet? Salty or cheesy? Dry or wet? Hot or cold? Think of foods with similar characteristics.

A similar approach, called "fading," makes minute changes to an accepted food, like adding a small amount of peach yogurt to vanilla yogurt and gradually increasing the peach. Think of fading as making small changes to one food, while chaining links one food to another through common properties like crunchy texture.

Cognitive Bridges

For the child with EPE, small differences in foods can scare him, so the goal is to help him see the similarities. Remember "chicken-steak"? Giving your child that connection to a food he is familiar with eases him into learning about a new food. You might say: **"This is a cheese-cracker. It tastes like cheese but is crunchy like your other crackers."** Or **"This is pasta like your spaghetti. It's spaghetti-bowties!"** Or **"You know how I make those zucchini muffins? These are zucchini-carrot muffins."** Or **"Did you know bunny-boo loves carrots?"**

The last example is a context clue that's a little more fun: a child fixated on bunnies, for example, may be curious about carrots if she learns that bunnies like carrots. One nonverbal child with autism began eating dog food out of the dog's bowl, exasperating his mother. Jenny suggested serving the family food from an identical dog bowl at the table. Why not? The child was eating ten new foods within a few days, and soon enough was using a regular plate. This is an example of a cognitive bridge—the visual of the bowl.

Taste Bridges

If a food doesn't taste good, children are unlikely to come back for more. As previously stated, nutrition doesn't motivate the vast majority of children; having a pleasurable experience is their goal. But children can learn to find more foods that taste good. Start with flavors your child enjoys: savory, salty, sweet, sour, or tart. Build a repertoire of foods with those flavors that you can rotate into eating opportunities.

Condiment Bridges

Parents often express a reluctance to serve sauces and dips, worrying the child won't learn to eat foods plain, or about the health implications of fat, sugar, or salt. Think of ketchup and dips as training wheels; you probably won't have a teenager pouring ketchup on rice or corn on the cob (but you'll survive if you do). Many adults prefer steak with steak sauce, or love the punch of added Tabasco, salt, pepper, or other toppings. Children should be allowed the same option.

Condiments help children learn to like new foods. If a child likes chicken with ketchup, she may enjoy other meats (or potatoes) with ketchup. For tougher or dry foods like meats, dips and sauces add moisture, making them easier to manage. Have a variety of options, such as ketchup, ranch dressing, homemade honey-mustard dressing, or hot sauce, on the table at meals and snacks.

Sweet Bridges

Adding some sweetness makes many foods more palatable, especially when the food is naturally bitter, like broccoli or brussels sprouts. While white sugar is fine, there are alternatives that provide sweetness along with some nutritional benefits. Honey, coconut nectar, agave nectar, and molasses are a few you can try. Applesauce is good for baking and can replace up to half the sugar in a cake recipe, or be added to complete recipes for additional sweetness, like in pancakes. A ripe banana can stand in for sugar when you're baking at home or can sweeten a pudding. Blend frozen bananas with other ingredients into a smoothie. Sweet bridges offer opportunities to sample new flavors and textures.

Liquid Bridges

Many children are less particular about liquids than solid foods. Using juices, nectars, or smoothies to introduce flavors may be easier than introducing a flavor in its whole form. Here are some ideas:

- If your child enjoys apple juice, try serving half applesauce, half apple juice in a fun cup with a straw.

- Mix apple juice with a little yogurt and freeze it in ice-cube trays with toothpicks, or a frozen pop mold, for a frozen treat.

- For the child who enjoys orange juice, make orange smoothies.

- Try a juicer so your child can see where orange juice comes from; he might suck the juice straight from the orange.

- Try soy-based fruit drinks that are the consistency of milk but come in a variety of flavors, providing more protein and nutritionally dense calories than juice.

- Serve smooth soups like tomato, potato-leek, or butternut squash in a cup—your child may not eat soup with a spoon, but he may drink it!

- Offer Yo-J (orange juice and yogurt blend) or drinkable yogurt (mix it into milk if it is an accepted drink, and gradually increase the amount).

For the child who only drinks water or plain milk, ease into flavor using the "fading" method mentioned earlier. Changing the color may be the place you start. Introduce food coloring (natural food dye if you prefer) that your child can drip into water or milk. You can talk about the colors when you mix them. After assuring her it won't taste different, you can see if she wants to try her green water. If your child happily drinks the colored water, next time see if she's up for adding flavored ice cubes. Mix half water and half juice (try white grape juice if you think colored ice will upset her), make small ice cubes, and let her add one to her water. The first few sips won't taste any different, but as the ice melts, her water will have a slightly different taste. If it's not a positive experience, scoop out the ice cube or dump it out and get her clean water. The last thing you want is to ruin a safe drink. Be cautious with milk if it's a major source of nutrition.

The Child Who Resists Drinking

Liquids can bridge to new flavors—unless your child doesn't like to drink! Children can drink different amounts and be healthy. Some children (particularly those with a history of aspirating or of trouble with liquids) resist drinking or don't seem to drink enough and may have dark yellow or concentrated urine or chronic constipation. (Dehydration contributes to constipation.) Avoid the temptation to push liquids. Just like with eating, pressuring a child to drink can backfire. Think about your child's sensory preferences or oral motor weaknesses as you optimize fluid intake. Could you provide liquids in a more manageable or appealing way?

- For the child who prefers strong input, consider tart juices like cranberry or pomegranate, add lime or lemon juice to drinks, or mix juice with sparkling water.

- If liquid intake is so low as to cause problems and your child prefers flavored drinks (MiO water enhancers, Hansen's Natural Fruit Stix, or watered-down juices), you may offer them between meals, but be careful not to spoil appetite. (Ideally you are offering only water between eating opportunities.)

- Try a different cup, a sports bottle, or a straw cup. One mom was amazed when her son happily drank water from a fancy glass with a lemon slice brought by a waitress.

- Let your child use the fridge water dispenser or invest in a water cooler they can work themselves. More control may motivate drinking and paying attention to subtle thirst cues.

- Keep cups where kids can reach them easily; maybe in a little tub near the cooler.

- Some children with oral motor problems dislike thin liquids because they flow too quickly backward in the mouth. Try slightly thicker milk or fruit nectars that are easier to swallow. A registered pediatric dietitian can suggest food-based thickeners.

- Try smoothies made with ice cubes, juice, or frozen fruits.

- Make afternoon snack time a tea party with a preferred liquid.

- Boost liquid intake with fruits such as watermelon or cut-up grapes. Fruits have high water content as well as fiber.

- Try decaf fruit teas, such as lemon or berry flavor, served warm or cold. Add honey or sugar if needed. Kids can enjoy iced tea in summer too.

- Serve shaved or crushed ice in a dish or cup with a spoon; you can pour some juice over or just let them eat the ice.

- Try flavored milk: chocolate, strawberry, or vanilla, or flavored milk straws.

- Offer Jell-O, frozen pops, or sorbets and sherbets for dessert.

- Serve canned fruit or fruit cups in 100 percent juice and let your child drink the juice.

Improving oral motor control or finding the right cup (see our "Resources" page online, http://www.newharbinger.com/31106) with an experienced speech-language pathologist's help can do wonders for your child's willingness to drink.

Your Child's Choice May Be a Bridge

Some parents new to the division of responsibility (your job: what, when, and where; your child's job: whether and how much) think that if their job is to decide what to serve, they can't let the child make any decisions or suggestions. We often hear, "What if my child asks for something I'd let him have anyway?" There is room for flexibility, and sometimes when a child can choose or have some say, it can motivate or bridge to a new food. As long as you are generally deciding what the options are, it's not only okay but respectful to take your child's choices into account, helping her feel more in control and less anxious. Older children who may be used to getting their own snacks and even meals will appreciate being included in menu planning. Say: **"Would you like Ritz or Cheez-Its with snack?"** Or **"Would you like your banana cut up or whole?"** Or **"Would you like blueberries or strawberries in your smoothie?"**

If your child suggests a food for a meal or snack, and you are okay with it, you can allow that. For example, if she says, "Mom, can we have rice with the chicken tonight?" say: **"Good idea, I'll make rice."** Otherwise, you might say something like: **"We had rice last night— tonight we are having noodles—do you want straight or curly ones?"** If she can't decide, or you are getting sucked into negotiating, postpone offering choices for now.

Sweets and Treats

We've already covered serving dessert with the meal. Part two of helping your child learn to manage high-interest foods is the "treat snack." It looks like this: one or two times a week, serve a snack where a treat or high-interest food is included, and let him eat as much as he wants. When a child routinely sneaks foods like candy or cookies, bringing them into the meal and snack rotation helps him learn to manage those foods. This is done by offering one serving as a dessert with a meal, and occasionally a plate of cookies for snack.

For example: after school, make his favorite chocolate pudding together and let him lick the spoon or bowl. Sit down and enjoy the snack with milk, perhaps also with a favorite fruit so he has the option of getting a little more balance. If the snack food is mostly carbs, like candy, try to offer some fat and protein as well (perhaps milk with at least some fat in it).

It can be scary, because your child may eat lots of the treat snack initially—rarely, he may eat so much that he even makes himself sick. However, hovering and warning him not to eat too much may make him anxious and want more (remember, kids like to do the opposite of what parents want). If you can learn to tolerate his eating more than you may feel comfortable with, then in time, you should see your child eat less of the high-interest foods, and ask for those foods less often.

Putting Foods Away

If your child has certain foods he pesters you for, like a cracker, granola bar, cheese stick, or applesauce pouch, keeping them out of sight can decrease his pestering. (Note: The occasional sneaking of food is normal in childhood.) Many kids who see cookies or a favorite food will ask for it whether they are hungry or not, if it is a safe food or if they are bored. Keeping treats in a cupboard and serving them at regular intervals helps children learn to incorporate them into a balanced diet.

Special Circumstances

What if your child doesn't eat well at school or gets sick, or you have religious or dietary restrictions? You can support his eating even in the face of challenges.

Packed Meals

If you are trying to pack more of a variety of foods, but your child's lunch is coming back day after day untouched, honor your need to nurture and provide. It's all right, particularly in the beginning, to pack foods your child is very likely to eat. Rotate in choices from his "safe" list if you can, or include small amounts of more challenging foods. Investigate for other barriers:

- How much time does your child have to eat?

- Can he open containers on his own?

- Is temperature an issue? Can you freeze yogurt tubes so they are cold at lunchtime?

- Is lunch right before recess, so he's eager to get outside to maximize playtime?

- Is he eating in his snowsuit or carrying gloves or a hat that get in his way?

- Are adults or other children pressuring him to eat?

Monitor how things are going and move at his pace. One typically picky child who ate a fair variety was anxious when his family moved overseas, refusing anything for lunch at his new kindergarten other than peanut butter and jelly. For the first six weeks, that's what his mom packed, and as he learned more of the language and made some friends, and his general anxiety decreased, she added more variety.

Remember not to ask about lunch or look in his lunchbox first thing. If he isn't eating much at lunch for whatever reason, be ready with a filling and accepted snack right after school, when he may be hungry.

When Your Child Is Sick

When a child with EPE is sick with a stomach bug or head cold, parents are sometimes told they still have to get the same number of bites or ounces in "no matter what." Many have shared with us how tough it is on both them and their children to follow this advice.

> **Food for Thought:** When you are sick, does your appetite change? Do you want to eat more or less? Does it depend on if it's a cold or a stomach virus?

If your child is unwell, respond to her needs. Allow her to lick frozen pops or nibble on Jell-O all day, or sip broth from a thermos in bed. Relax your structure to meet her needs (and yours). Check in with your child's health care provider during illnesses. Have faith that as she gets better, you and she can get back on track with the steps, even if it takes a few days: in our experience, this is almost always what happens.

Meal Planning with Restrictions

When a child is struggling, whether it is with stomach issues, constipation, or behavioral or learning problems, some parents consider dietary interventions as part of treatment. The research we have seen on dietary interventions in general is unclear, and parents' experiences are mixed. Specific dietary interventions are beyond the scope of this book, but if you research and choose to pursue a specialized diet, having STEPS+ in place will be key to the success of the trial, which should usually last a minimum of three to six months. Consider that pursuing elimination diets while a child is still struggling with eating can worsen power struggles and appetite. Often a child's favorites are the first to go: macaroni and cheese, pastas, breads, and milk.

Taking away safe foods can make him more anxious and cause regression.

An elimination diet means new ways of cooking, meal planning, and other tasks. Be kind with yourself through the process, and ask for help and support. Here are some tips to help you through:

- Focus on what your child *can* eat.

- Have a positive attitude. Stick with the other steps. Avoid acting on the principle that "Because he can't have so many things, I'll let him have treats whenever he asks."

- If possible, the whole family should follow the plan. Serving your child his special foods while you graze on other foods isn't very supportive. Consider the child's dietary restrictions without being too obvious, while meeting the needs of others. (Can a sibling enjoy cheese pizza out with friends?)

- Be matter-of-fact about what your child can or can't eat. Don't call it a "diet."

- Link it back to how your child feels. Say: **"Regular milk makes your tummy hurt. Let's try this milk today."**

- Make gradual changes using fading or chaining, described in "Building Bridges to New Foods" earlier in this chapter.

- Find safe alternatives for accepted foods (like gluten-free).

- Keep the structure, saying no to requests for food between eating opportunities but allowing water. Continue to enjoy family meals.

With elimination diets, we wonder if success is due more to the removal of certain foods or more to the parents' increased attention to overall balance, preparing meals, and eating together. If it helps (that is, your child is happier and healthier), the "why" might not matter.

Religious Considerations

If your family's eating habits follow a religious code, hopefully you have a community that shares your eating style. In addition to the tips given for approaching restrictions, focus on and celebrate the cultural and family connections and the reasons behind the food rules. For example, discuss how it makes you feel closer to God and how this is important for your family.

Some clients have difficulty with religious requirements, such as menu planning or meeting nutrition needs while keeping kosher, honoring the Sabbath, or fasting. If your child is small or doesn't deal well with low blood-sugar levels, or if going without food is scary for him, expecting him to fast may be too much. Explore concerns with your religious leaders and with your conscience, and seek out support.

At this point, you've tackled most of the steps, including specific ideas about how to put both familiar and new foods on the table to support your child's eating, keeping his challenges and preferences in mind. The next chapter will guide you in helping your child overcome oral motor or sensory challenges in particular, including determining whether and when it's time to seek an evaluation or therapy.

CHAPTER 8

Step 5: Build Skills

If your child has oral motor or sensory challenges, ways of introducing foods that may be fine for other children may not meet your child's needs. This chapter is designed to help you help your child build skills and increase the variety of foods he eats. It's divided into two sections. The first section shares specific ideas for preparing and presenting foods, including use of plates, utensils, and cups. We'll also explore ways to offer opportunities for your child to build oral motor stability and coordination and sensory awareness, and increase his familiarity and comfort with a variety of foods so he can come to the table more prepared to eat the foods you serve.

The second section focuses on what to do if these tips, and the STEPS+ program, don't feel like enough, and you wonder if it's time for an evaluation or therapy. You may have just gotten a therapy referral, or perhaps realized your child's current therapy is wrong for your family. This section touches on different approaches, who provides therapy, how to find the right therapist or program, and how to know if therapy may be making things worse. Whether or not your path leads to formal therapy, you can help your child build skills at home.

Building Skills and Familiarity

The way food is presented, including the shape, utensils, or how it is served, can make that subtle and unpredictable difference as to how your child feels about a food, and her willingness to try it. We'll start with ideas for presenting a wide variety of foods in different ways, expanding on what you learned in chapter 7.

Self-Feeding Skills

Presenting foods in new or different ways supports self-feeding, particularly if your child has a negative association with spoons, certain plates, or therapy tasks. You can try these strategies if there are oral motor or sensory concerns and even if your child is just learning or has a general developmental delay:

- Allow your child to eat with his hands or a combination of hands and utensils.

- Use two spoons; give your child a spoon to dip and explore with, while you feed him with another spoon. It shares the task and gives him some control. Try loading one spoon and handing it to him, or trade off.

- Present a non-spoon dipper such as a wooden craft stick, chopsticks, or a commercial toddler dipper such as the Gerber Lil' Dipper.

- Try the DuoSpoon (developed by Marsha Dunn Klein): both ends of this flexible, bumpy spoon provide different sensory input during mouth exploration and eating. The bowl part of the spoon is very shallow—great for beginning eaters and children working on eating skills.

- Food presented on a utensil (or nonutensil) such as a large wooden spoon, a whisk, or a flat plastic lid can spark curiosity.

- For children able to use them safely, try toothpicks in various colors and shapes—swords, animal-topped picks, and so on. Use them to spear noodles or pieces of veggies from soups, or to pick up chunks of melon or chicken.

- Older kids can thread foods like cut-up fruit or cheese (or anything that will stay on) onto sticks or skewers. One mom watched in wonder while her six-year-old who "never eats meat" ate three chicken satay skewers at a buffet.

- Show your child how to use chopsticks—some Asian restaurants provide connectors to help your child get the hang of it. "Trainer" chopsticks with fun shapes and designs are also available in stores.

- Try a favorite (nontoxic) toy to dip into foods, like those popular squeaky giraffes or chewable jewelry.

- Hard, crunchy foods such as large crackers can be used to scoop food and help a spoon-averse child realize that food is separate from the spoon.

- Try plates with compartments so foods don't touch. Younger children may like patterns or characters. For older children, there are plain plates similar to cafeteria trays. You can also use a small plate and a few small bowls that they can serve into.

- Let the struggle over manners go for now. If it's enjoyable for everyone, make manners fun and pressure free with a weekly "fancy night" where you put out nice dishes and talk with accents, sip drinks with pinkies extended, and practice using silverware.

Drinking Skills

Drinking from straws and open cups may come later for kids with oral motor delays. Some children have trouble giving up the bottle, or find drinking from a transitional or sippy cup difficult. The goal is drinking in a developmentally appropriate way. Straws are a great way for kids to drink independently and are preferable to sippy cups due to the different shape and more mature sucking pattern needed. Cups with straws also minimize spills and are convenient away from home. One of Jenny's favorites for children who are having trouble with straws is a cup with a one-way valve straw, like Ark's Cip-Kup, a flexible, lidded cup that helps children learn to suck. The adult can even squeeze gently until a little fluid moves up into the straw and into the child's mouth, or you can help her squeeze. The fluid stays in the straw due to the valve, reducing frustration when she can't maintain suction and loses the fluid over and over. This is not a necessary step for typically developing children, but some children benefit from a little assistance early in the process.

Other specialized cups, some developed for therapeutic use, include:

- DOIDY cup: the unique slant teaches children to drink from a rim and not a spout.

- Lollacup: a two-handled cup with a weighted, valve-free straw that anchors in the liquid so the child can drink even when the cup is tilted.

- Playtex Coolster Tumbler: insulated and shaped like a to-go coffee cup; taking the valve out creates the effect of an open cup without so much spillage.

- Playtex First Lil' Gripper Straw Trainer Cup: squeezable cup helps parents teach children how to drink through a straw.

Older kids may prefer a grown-up cup or a fancy straw. Watch out for some of the sippy cups with strong valves that require a strong suck—they can make an already difficult task even harder. As your child works to move beyond the sippy cup or bottle, here are some ways to help her:

- Start by bringing the sippy cup or bottle to the table during meals and snacks and out of circulation during laps around the house.

- Introduce a new sippy or straw cup.

- Switch out the lids so that they are mismatched, adding interest and conversation; say: **"Spiderman likes having a Superman lid!"**

- Offer beverages at meals in both the favored cup and an open cup so your child can practice, or let her practice taking sips from your cup with assistance as she learns.

One mom shared that her young son would find family members' cups sitting around the house and then dump them on himself, trying to drink. He didn't have the hand and arm control to hold the cup steady at the correct angle, and Mom was tired of changing his clothes three times a day! Jenny suggested a weighted, two-handled cup with an insert lid, with a small hole for drinking. The extra weight gave him more awareness in (and of) his arms, which allowed him to drink and put the cup down without spilling (the weighted bottom also helped it stand upright). Remarkably, after a week or so of drinking from this cup, he figured out how to drink from other cups—and he was no longer tossing Dad's iced tea!

Chewing Skills

Children with poor chewing skills tend to select foods for ease of chewing (among other qualities like flavor or visual appeal), preferring soft foods that stick together when mashed and don't require grinding: cereal bars, macaroni and cheese, hash browns, yogurt, chicken nuggets—these are a few of their favorite things! Many of these children have already been in feeding therapies, often with a sensory focus. If a child can't chew more complex textures, it may look as if the problem is sensory or texture aversion; a chewing deficit can go undetected.

Learning to chew is critical for the struggling child. Jenny recommends chewing aids for many children, with great results. (Some therapists recommend against them, but we don't think it's necessary to take any tools out of your toolkit if your child accepts them.) When babies begin to strengthen jaw and tongue muscles, they aren't chewing on food—they are chewing on toys, their fingers, pacifiers, parents' fingers, or clothes. Many children who don't chew well have a history of limited mouthing as infants. A parent might note, "She never put anything in her mouth, while her twin chewed on my fingers and anything she could reach all the time!"

Moving something solid around in their mouths knowing that they won't have to swallow gives many children confidence to explore and gain strength and coordination safely. Your child may not feel safe putting a carrot in his mouth, but will readily chew on a rubber chewing stick. The use of such aids as Chewy Tubes, Thera-Tubing, NUK brushes, or Tri-Chews allows children to go back to mouthing, critical for learning how to chew and handle different textures.

Using Chewing Aids

If you think your child might benefit from chewing aids, a speech-language pathologist can show you where they are placed in the mouth and how to use them. If you don't have a therapist or want to try them at home, your child still benefits if he chews on these at all. If there is a lot of strengthening to be done, it's best not to use chewing aids while your child is eating, as he can get fatigued and not chew as well on the food, decreasing intake. Here are some ideas for incorporating chewing aids:

- Use them to dip favored foods like yogurts, peanut butter, marshmallow fluff, or purees.

- Offer them between mealtimes or in the tub (if that's a fun time) or in front of the mirror.

- Model chewing on the tube and let your child imitate you. Show her how to place it perpendicular to her teeth.

- A younger child might enjoy pretending she's a dog hanging on to a bone with her teeth while you gently try to tug it out.

Another benefit to using a tool for building chewing skills is that it helps a child accept nonfood items in his mouth. Struggles around brushing teeth are a prime complaint for parents of children with oral aversions, and handling the sensation of something in his mouth is the first step to making tooth brushing possible and more pleasant. In fact, many strategies for building chewing skills can be adapted to tooth brushing: for example, use two toothbrushes and let your child help while you "double-check," or let him play with a toothbrush in the tub. Giving a cue for the beginning and ending of the brushing— for example, **"Three zooms and I'm done…zoom, zoom, zoom!"**— will help him feel less anxious.

Building Sensory Skills with Nonfood Sensory Play

Digging in dirt, splashing in water, scooping and pouring sand, or smearing finger paint may be one child's heaven and another child's nightmare: children have a broad range of sensory temperaments, and it affects how they learn to eat. From the first introduction of solid foods, most infants touch and explore food to familiarize themselves with the texture. By looking and touching, infants get clues about what they will need to do with food in their mouths. Some infants don't seek, and even actively avoid the sensations and miss out. For some toddlers and children with sensory problems and EPE, encouraging a return to exploratory play with different textures increases comfort with and tolerance for different sensations, and they grow more comfortable with a variety of foods. Here are some ideas for sensory and exploratory play:

- Fill a large bin with dried lentils or rice and bury items for your child to find.

- Put oats in a large baking dish with sides and let your child measure, scoop, and play.

- Let your child finger paint or play with bath foams or bubbles in the tub.

- Let your child use her hands to scoop birdseed into the feeder.

There are dozens of online resources dedicated to sensory play. When sensory problems are a major obstacle, occupational therapy has helped many children; it is described in the second half of this chapter.

Food for Thought: Would you eat something you wouldn't touch with your hands?

Building Familiarity Outside of Therapy and Mealtimes

Family meals at the table are the ultimate goal. However, if the table has become a negative space, your child might need a fresh start. Finding ways to interact with food without pressure can change negative associations into positive ones. Removing the expectation of eating goes a long way toward reducing perceived pressure and can help your child become less wary and more familiar with different foods.

Play with Your Food

We offer activities that involve interacting with or tasting foods with a word of caution. Playing a game with the agenda of increasing your child's comfort with food can backfire if she is easily overwhelmed or feels pressured by the activity. One mom shared that when she tried to have her child paint with pudding, he had a full-on tantrum. At the first sign of anxiety or resistance, let it go and move on to an activity she enjoys. If you have more than one child, involve your other children and focus on together time, so your child with EPE doesn't feel singled out and pressured. You might also wait until you have the rest of the steps in place. Here are some ideas for fun with food:

- Go outside with a marshmallow shooter and see how far they go. Talk about what lucky bird or squirrel might get to nibble one.

- Feed ducks, or feed pretend fish in a bathtub or large bowl.

- Build a gingerbread house with all the candy trimmings.

- Pull out your spices for a guessing game. Ask your child to close her eyes and offer her a sniff of vanilla or oregano. See if she can tell the difference. (Careful! Sniffing cinnamon can sting.) Ask if it smells like cake or pizza.

- Have your child help label and organize the pantry or spice rack. Kids often love label makers, or making labels themselves.

- Make crumbs for a coating or piecrust; have your child put crackers in a baggie and roll them out with a rolling pin or crush them with her hands.

- For children who enjoy craft projects, gather colorful condiments such as ketchup, mustard, mayonnaise, caramel topping, chocolate syrup, marshmallow fluff, or peanut butter and have them create a piece of art. Add in some safe foods (Goldfish crackers) along with new ones (raisins), and you might see your child nibble while she works.

- Make stamps out of potatoes or limes and use them to make wrapping paper or stationery.

- Draw basic faces on paper plates and use food to fill in hair, eyes, mouth, and so on.

- Spear small pieces of food with toothpicks or pick them up with tongs: pick up and drop new foods onto a target drawn on construction paper for a quick and easy interaction.

- Make snow ice cream. In a big bowl, combine 4 cups of fresh snow, 1/2 cup of heavy cream, 1/4 cup of sugar, and, if you like, 1/2 teaspoon of vanilla. Mix with a wooden spoon.

Look online for other suggestions; one list we particularly like is on Marsha Dunn Klein's Mealtime Notions website.

Head to the Store

Going to an unfamiliar grocery store helps you to consider items you may not have ever offered. Take your child along with you for an adventure into unknown territory. He can help you find things you always buy, as well as point out intriguing items—he might surprise you! Have him help you count or weigh fruit, or help him feel capable by asking him, for example, to find and bring you three oranges. One father described how his three-year-old son enthusiastically chose foods once it occurred to him to let his son out of the cart: "He was face to face with more choices, and could get his hands on more things."

Exercise: Try to replace three items on your grocery list with new ones. For example, if you always buy fresh green beans, try white beans, canned green beans, or zucchini.

Research Recipes Together

Pull out your best-loved cookbooks and let your child select a recipe to make together. Read off the list of ingredients or let her read them to you. Show her pictures, or go online so she can see the end result. Make an effort to stay calm during this process as your child eliminates recipes or if she settles on a known quantity like pancakes.

Look for simple recipes or head to the bookstore or library for kids' cookbooks. Older children can menu plan and even prepare simple family meals, but they don't have to eat what they make. Avoid saying, "You chose it, at least try it!" And thank your child for cooking!

The process of choosing, gathering ingredients, and helping to cook provides a real-world, developmentally true way for your child to learn about foods, increase familiarity with different foods, and have good times with you. One dad cooked meals with a fan in the kitchen to help ease his daughter's sensitivity to smells, and they enjoyed their time together while she handled and learned about different foods. If your child doesn't want to help, don't push, but do keep offering. Some kids like helping in the kitchen and others don't.

Exercise: Take pictures of meals or snacks your child helped prepare. Note what you liked and what you might change next time. Build a family recipe book. Let your child make up funny names; applesauce might be "Amy's Awesome-sauce."

Garden Variety

Children are more likely to try and eat foods they helped grow or prepare, but there's no guarantee. As always, don't pressure your child or try to make him eat.

- Grow something—anything—even one of those upside-down tomato plants.

- Set up a window herb garden or a small garden plot in your yard. It doesn't matter so much if you have a green thumb; the process of planning, planting, nurturing, and finally harvesting familiarizes your child with the foods.

- Cut a sprouted potato in half and have your child put it cut-end down in a shallow dish near a window with a half-inch of water. He can change the water every few days and watch it grow.

- Visit a peach or apple orchard or berry farm and pick fruit as a family.

If you don't have the desire, time, space, or energy to garden, head to a farmer's market or a grocery store that offers samples. Go during a planned snack or mealtime, when your child might be hungry, and bring some safe food with you. Have no expectations, but let him check out the options. Give him a few dollars to spend on what he chooses, and be ready to buy something that your skeptical side doesn't think he will eat.

Jenny and a colleague led a social-skills group centered on gardening for children with mild autism. It was amazing to watch the kids dig, make a scarecrow, and harvest. When they baked carrot muffins and made onion dip from the vegetables they grew to sell to their parents, one boy decided he had to try a muffin before the sale. His mom gaped as he took a huge bite. Thus began a beautiful relationship with carrots. You too can garden or cook, maybe even "selling" the final product to a willing friend.

Addressing Challenges

A big part of our work is brainstorming solutions to common obstacles. This section reviews some of these solutions, such as removing distractions, food preparation for kids with oral motor or sensory challenges, helping children feed and serve themselves, and using special gear. We also address rarer problems like pocketing (or cheeking) food and overstuffing.

Weaning Off Distractions

Many families are accustomed to relying on distractions to get one or two more bites in. Some children only eat in front of a screen, and many therapy programs introduce TV, toys, iPads, and so on to reward a child for taking bites. This is external motivation, and we believe it is counterproductive. Distractions almost always "work" in the short term to get a few bites in—and that's why weaning off them feels scary. But distractions don't teach children to eat. Zoning out or dissociating from an uncomfortable feeding situation actually makes your child eat less in the long run because it interferes with her ability to tune in to her appetite.

Pleasant, low-anxiety family meals allow for loving interactions, and socializing can replace the device. Sitting at the table at a family meal *without a device* (and with no pressure to eat) will be new for your child; he may protest. Here are some approaches to weaning off screens and toys:

- Pick one device-free meal or snack a day, and work your way up. If your child is old enough, you might let him choose. You might say: **"Sally, I was so happy to have you sitting with us last night at dinner! You are so much fun to talk to. Let's eat breakfast together without the iPad so we can hear each other."**

- Start the meal without the screen, and don't get it until your child asks. You might then say something like: **"I really like talking to you without the iPad noise! Tell me about your day before we turn it on."** Or **"The battery is low; let's start without the Kindle while it charges."**

- Consider having no screen for the first ten minutes and then allowing it. If you don't bring out the device, does your child even notice? Your older child may also choose to start or end meals with five minutes of screen time as a transition.

- Instead of turning on the device, have a snack while you play a card game or do a puzzle together, taking the focus off eating and putting it on together time.

- Turn off *your* distractions! Turn off the phone, or leave it in another room so you aren't tempted. When you look at it, your child will want to also.

- Use a similar approach with books or toys. Say: **"I know we used to let you play during meals, but we're doing things differently. The table is now for food and talking, not toys."**

- With older children, talk about changing expectations away from meal and snack times. Ask them for ideas to reach your goals.

The first time you try a meal without a device, you may want to bring it back when your child becomes anxious so he doesn't get too upset. Try again when you feel ready.

Other distractions include dangling legs, which can tempt your child to fidget and kick; eating in a moving car; or too much visual stimulation. Here are some tips to address these:

- Sitting with supported posture reduces sitting fatigue and improves oral motor efficiency. Feeling more secure and grounded helps your child focus on signals from his body. Find a chair with a footrest, like the Tripp Trapp (or similar brand) with built-in, adjustable footrests. Or make your own footrest with a sturdy stool or box.

- Avoid eating in a moving car. In addition to the choking hazard, the distraction makes many children eat less. Some children may eat more in cars if they are used to eating only when distracted, or if the car is the one place where they can eat without pressure or attention. Phase out this ultimately unhelpful crutch as the table becomes less stressful.

- Simplify décor. Avoid crazy placemats, crayons, sparkly plates, striped napkins, and candelabras if your child is overwhelmed by visual stimulation.

Transitioning to Self-Feeding

Some therapy protocols insist on the parent feeding every bite, even after the child is able to feed herself. If you are stuck feeding a child who is able to work toward feeding herself, this is frustrating—for you and your child! The goal for your child who is transitioning to self-feeding is similar to that of the Montessori style of education: "Help me do it myself!" Here are some tips that can help you both make the transition:

- Cut her food into strips rather than pieces, so she can hold it easily and take bites.

- Spear her food onto a fork, or preload spoons, to make eating less frustrating. Keep two of each utensil handy to avoid battles.

- Try bowls or plates with tall sides to scoop against, or with suction cups to keep from sliding.

- Some children dislike messy fingers so much that they insist on being spoon-fed. Place a damp washcloth nearby so you can help your child wipe her hands when she wants. As she is able, teach her to wipe her own hands. This empowers her to cope on her own. (If she's not upset by messy hands or food on her chin, leave it until she's done. Wiping or scooping food off the chin with a spoon distracts and upsets some children.)

If you have concerns about your child's progress or skills with self-feeding, an occupational therapist can help, particularly if your child needs adaptive gear to do it herself.

Dealing with Pocketing or Cheeking Food

When kids keep food in their cheeks, you may wonder if they are being naughty, or saving food for later. Pocketing food increases choking risk and also gets in the way of eating and intake: if there is food in Johnny's mouth already, it is harder for him to go on to the next bite. Some children pocket food as a way to keep others from putting more in, and the behavior usually resolves on its own when pressure is removed. However, most children who pocket don't sense it is happening or don't know how to keep it from happening. A small mirror at the table can help your child become more aware of his mouth. Introduce the mirror before a meal and explain that you are going to do "cheek checks." You might say: **"This mirror is for you. We can look in your mouth and do a cheek check to see if it is clean. If it isn't, that means you need to swallow. If you need a drink to help you, here it is. If you want to spit it out, that's fine too."** He can help hold the mirror and look for food. Make sure he has a drink he can use to clear his mouth. Many children don't have the skills to get all the food from their cheeks once it gets stuck there. The drink washes it down.

Overstuffing Food

Remember the sensorimotor loop from chapter 2? The sensory system tells the motor system what is happening so the mouth can respond appropriately. When the sensory system has a glitch, over-stuffing can result: your child doesn't feel the bread in his mouth, so he puts more in until he *can* feel it. The problem with overstuffing is that once the mouth is that full, there is little room to move the tongue and food around to mix with saliva and chew. This makes swallowing almost impossible, and the whole mouthful is spit out. "Waking up" his mouth (alerting his system) to get ready for the meal can decrease overstuffing. Try the following:

- Offer a tart or ice-cold drink (lemonade or cranberry juice).

- Hand your child a vibrating toothbrush to play with in his mouth just before a meal.

- Keep a small bowl of crunchy or cold foods at the table (pretzel sticks, frozen peas, even ice chips).

- Some children with developmental delays learn to avoid over-stuffing through a visual reminder made with clip art or real pictures of the child for each step: 1) "I take a bite"; 2) "I chew and swallow"; 3) "My mouth is clean"; and 4) "I take another bite." This can be a useful transitional tool.

These tips are not necessary for the majority of children with EPE, and they can increase attention and therefore pressure. However, for the child with more significant sensory or oral motor problems, or who accepts them without resistance, they can help start a meal off right.

Still Gagging

If your steps are in place and your child is still gagging, there is likely something else going on. Anxiety can play a major role, so be sure to review chapter 4 on pressure. If you feel anxiety isn't the issue, and your child wants to swallow but can't without gagging, his system may not be in sync, as with overstuffing. He may become fatigued before the food is properly chewed, swallowing too early, which results in gagging. If tongue movement is not well coordinated—even if he can move his tongue without food—adding food complicates matters because of the sensory input and movement of the pieces. He may lose bits of food in the back or sides of his mouth, causing gagging. If you're still concerned, it may be time to bring in someone experienced with sensorimotor delays.

Investigating Therapy Options

Parents have many responses when a child's physician or teacher recommends an evaluation. They may feel hopeful, embarrassed, or resentful, or they may not want to expose their child to teasing or scrutiny. This section highlights important aspects to consider, from deciding if you want to pursue therapy to getting a diagnosis and setting goals.

How Do You Know If Your Child Needs an Evaluation?

In chapter 2, we discussed how hard it can be to differentiate a normal variation of oral motor and feeding skills from a problem that might benefit from professional help. Many suggested diagnostic criteria for feeding problems include aspects of normal development, or of development that is delayed but progressing. Any of the following problems in your child warrants evaluation:

- She is losing weight.

- She is not gaining weight appropriately.

- She has evidence of swallowing difficulties like lung infections from getting food or liquids in her lungs (aspirating).

- She frequently gags or vomits.

- She is unable to get beyond baby foods or purees by fifteen months of age, provided that appropriate foods have been presented without pressure for at least three months.

- She appears upset or in pain when eating.

It boils down to this: if you feel as if you don't know what to do and need guidance, you may benefit from bringing your child to a therapist. A good feeding therapist is a diagnostician who can put together the pieces of the puzzle (your child's history and current issues, and how feeding is going) and synthesize the information to come up with a plan. If you don't want to pursue therapy right now, you can always reevaluate and do so in the future.

Who Provides Feeding Therapy?

A speech-language pathologist (SLP, also known as a speech therapist or ST) or an occupational therapist (OT) usually provides feeding therapy. Sometimes a psychologist or behavioral specialist (board-certified behavior analyst, or BCBA) will address feeding. While SLPs and OTs have master's level training, most feeding knowledge is acquired after graduate school in continuing education courses. We have learned (from parents) that what matters most is the therapist's knowledge, experience, and communication skills.

A speech-language pathologist specializing in feeding is trained to assess and treat deficits in oral motor skills as well as swallowing (dysphagia). SLPs are versed in child development, allowing them to treat your child in age-appropriate and developmentally supportive ways. Experienced SLPs working with feeding are also trained in sensory and motor development.

Occupational therapists provide therapy with a sensory focus, and they are expert at helping children achieve the fine and gross motor skills needed for self-feeding. Children learn through guided play and manipulation of their environment in ways that address the child's sensory challenges. Some OTs obtain additional training in swallowing and oral motor skills, which is not typically part of OT training. The occupational therapist can be most helpful for children sensitive to touch, with whole-body sensory differences, or who need help with self-feeding. Depending on your child's needs and the skill level of your feeding therapist, your child might benefit from coordinated care with both an OT and an SLP.

Building Your Team

Whomever you are working with, whether an OT or SLP alone or a feeding team, good communication among involved providers (dietitian, GI doctor, or pediatrician) is critical. If there is one provider you most trust and connect with, she or he may serve as a case manager of sorts, directing you to other providers that fit your needs. Don't forget, however, that your GI doctor or allergist may not have training in feeding and might give advice conflicting with the feeding therapy. Check in with your feeding therapist before making changes, and request that your providers communicate with one another. Keeping your own copies of relevant records in one binder helps ensure everyone's on the same page; when the note from the dietitian didn't get to the GI doc, you have a copy.

The Initial Evaluation

The first evaluation should allow time for parents (with the child out of earshot, if she is old enough to understand) to discuss and review concerns and history with the therapist, who has reviewed any notes before the visit. (Ask the therapist in advance what records and foods to bring.) An experienced SLP then observes your child's oral motor skills without food as well as how she chews, moves food around, swallows, and reacts to food. The therapist should then review findings and impressions with you and recommend any further testing or referrals. Ideally the initial visit lasts between one-and-a-half and two hours. Jenny, for example, offers sixty- to ninety-minute evaluations plus a thirty-minute phone follow-up to answer questions and review findings and recommendations.

The evaluation can yield insights that are themselves a relief. As one mom of a preschooler said, "If I only knew he *couldn't* eat that, I wouldn't have been so frustrated." She had been serving her son apple slices with the peel and was certain he was just acting up when he spit everything out after chewing. An assessment revealed that he couldn't chew in a rotary or circular pattern (which grinds food), leaving him unable to properly chew the peel. He liked the taste and kept trying, but was never able to swallow. During the evaluation, Jenny cut off the peel and sliced the apples thinly, and he chowed down. It opened this mom's eyes to how and why her child struggled with other foods as well. Feeling heard and gaining understanding can help with feelings of guilt and confusion, and may be the confidence boost you need to get back on track.

After a thorough history and evaluation, a decision can be made *with you* as to whether therapy is needed or wanted, what approach fits your family's needs, and how often sessions will occur. Having a supportive therapist is like having a net to catch you when you fall.

What Does Good Therapy Look Like?

Good therapy should be developmentally appropriate and support both you and your child. It should provide information and teach you to help your child at home. Therapists also help you see progress.

Developmentally Appropriate

Successful therapy considers your child's chronological and developmental age. That means matching activities with your child's age, interests, abilities, and temperament. When parents are told by therapists to place their nine-month-old baby in front of the TV for several hours a day to get him to eat, we are appalled. At the other end of the spectrum, an eleven-year-old isn't interested in painting with pudding while surrounded by pictures of cartoon characters.

Supportive of You and Your Child

Good therapy supports you as a parent, your child as his own person, and your needs as a family. Problem solving with input from you is a feeding therapist's bread and butter, including brainstorming about what types of foods to serve, how to tweak presentation, and helping you think creatively about meals. The therapist must have patience with you and your child. It isn't supportive if you feel as if your child is pushed to do more than he is ready for. We hear of parents who reluctantly agreed to let their toddler or preschooler work alone with a therapist, listening to their screaming child from the waiting room. It is not realistic to expect every child to be able to go with a stranger, especially without a transition. These children were pushed beyond what they were ready for, and progress is unlikely. Talk about anxiety!

You Become the Therapist

Your therapist should provide ideas and a model of how to interact with your child around food. Giving some direct intervention to a child and then passing it on to the parent is considered best practice in early intervention, which applies to feeding therapy. If your child will eat with the therapist but not with you, what's the point? Your child is with the therapist maybe one hour a week; what about the other 167?

Your therapist might model chewing on a Chewy Tube, and your child may imitate. Parent graduates of Jenny's STEPS program at the University of Texas–Dallas Callier Center for Communication Disorders said that having therapists model and teach them how to help their children with strengthening exercises or how to spit out food was most helpful. If your therapist isn't doing so, ask her to show you. Your therapist should interact with you as much as with your child, if not more.

Supporting you means that the therapist considers *your needs* as well. Do *you* feel pushed beyond your comfort level? This mom did: "I was scared to give up the purees, but my therapist kept telling me to with no explanation. I just kept giving purees. I never felt like I could tell her what was going on without being told I was doing it wrong. Our new therapist listens and we serve purees with some meals so I am reassured Henry is getting something." If you feel like *you* are being pushed, or threatened with scare tactics or feeding tubes, or you feel like you can't speak honestly with your therapist, it is not a working partnership.

Shows You What You Can't See on Your Own

When you watch your child not eat day in and day out, you get bogged down in it. The feeding therapist can point out successes you might not see. One mom shared that when the therapist pointed out how her son was better able to close his lips around a spoon, it helped her have faith in the process and avoid slipping back into insisting he eat.

How Long Will It Take?

At the start of feeding therapy, parents often ask how long it will take. While many children only need a few sessions of therapy with the parents supporting progress at home, other families need more intensive support. They may need to start with occupational therapy to help the child get comfortable around food, or get used to other tactile experiences. Direct feeding therapy can take many forms, but the intensity and duration depend on many factors. For example, a child who has never had anything by mouth will need more support than the child who is selective but eats. If the child has been in pressuring or anxiety-provoking therapies previously, it can take longer for her to regain trust before moving forward.

A Therapeutic Continuum

Many clients we work with who have stopped unsuccessful therapies are dismayed to find out that there are different approaches. They ask, "Why wasn't I told we had a choice?" This section is an introduction to those options, to help you make more informed decisions.

There are many therapeutic strategies focusing on sensory, oral motor, or behavioral aspects of eating. It's helpful to think of the range of therapies as a continuum: On one end, the feeder relies entirely on the child's internal motivation to eat. The idea is that the child will gain oral motor skills and familiarity with different foods in the course of daily living in a supportive environment of nonpressured, pleasant family meals. This is a valid approach for a great number of children, particularly if parents have good support and information.

Next along the continuum might be sensorimotor/play-based intervention with either a speech-language pathologist or an occupational therapist. Therapists may work directly with the child (sometimes for a short time or intermittently), but heavily target education to caregivers so that they learn to read the child's cues, allow the child to set the pace, and encourage autonomy and internal motivation. This would be most consistent with Jenny's therapeutic approach. A child who may progress over several months to years without therapy may make the same progress in a number of weeks with sensorimotor skills directly targeted.

Further along the continuum might be play or systematic desen-sitization therapies, which avoid outright pressure and aim to decrease anxiety and make therapy fun. This type of therapy aims to increase amounts eaten through positive reinforcement such as praise and external motivation, driven by the belief that children with EPE are unable to sense or tune in to signals of internal regulation. Foods are often preplated, and children perform tasks like blowing on or kissing foods to get them off a plate. It follows hierarchies of increasing comfort, with the child first tolerating a food nearby; then touching with a utensil, then a finger; then having the food touch the arms, face, lips, and so on. This is felt by some children as pressure, as it invites focused attention on food and the child, and it is less effective for children who are not motivated by praise or rewards.

Beyond this, more adult-directed therapy programs in outpatient clinics use positive reinforcement (toys or videos) as external motiva-tions and may promote ignoring children when they don't take bites. One step further includes day patient programs that use negative rein-forcement (such as escape extinction, where children aren't allowed to get out of taking a bite) and positive reinforcement (such as toys or videos).

Day programs and inpatient therapy programs most often use the applied behavioral analysis (ABA) model, also known as behavioral modification. This might include five to six meals a day where, after the parent is removed initially, the child is shown a video or given a toy when she takes a bite and is ignored when she doesn't. The focus is on volume, and purees are given from a spoon with little consider-ation for developmental stages, preferences, or self-feeding. This end of the continuum relies on external motivation and consistently over-rides internal motivation. The most extreme therapy has children restrained and force-fed—a practice we believe is *never* warranted. If a child is truly in nutritional crisis, we prefer gastric tube-feeding to force-feeding.

Increasingly we hear of psychologists working with children who have "failed" the above therapies. These children are introduced to "flooding" or "exposure therapies" with therapists, many of whom

194

have little training or understanding of the complex nature of feeding challenges and problems and who try to address them in a way similar to other anxieties. As we mentioned in chapter 4, we believe it best to address anxiety separately and that exposure therapies have the potential to intensify pressure and anxiety around eating.

STEPS+ Can Be Used with Some Therapies

Family meals, decreasing anxiety, and establishing a routine are helpful with almost all therapies. We often hear, "We don't pressure at home, but the OT at school wants to see if she can get him to eat more fruits and vegetables at snack." Or "The behaviorist who helped with potty training wants us to use the reward chart for his eating." The previously mentioned therapies that rely on external motivation and pressure are not consistent with STEPS+. The focus is still on getting the child to eat different or more food, often decreasing internal motivation and increasing anxiety and resistance. Children can work on oral motor exercises and the tips in this chapter as they are able, but generally if the child is also in behavioral therapies or even some of the desensitization therapies, progress will be undermined.

Finding a Good Fit

Because comprehensive training in this specialty is difficult to obtain, the skill and experience of individual therapists varies. You may have to do some legwork to find the right therapist for your family. For a list of questions to ask potential therapists and open a dialogue regarding training, experience, process, and approach, visit http://www.newharbinger.com/31106.

After reading this book, you should have a general understanding of which therapeutic approaches are compatible with STEPS+ if that's the way you decide to go. Your interaction with the therapist should indicate if she will be a good partner as you work to support internally motivated eating within your routine and meals, while avoiding pressure. If you still aren't sure whether a particular therapy program or therapist is a good match, ask prospective therapists for referrals or testimonials and talk to other parents who are clients. Ask an online support group for recommendations that may be more in line with the approach to feeding you want to pursue.

Keeping Therapy on Track

If you get a sinking feeling in your stomach before therapy, or if your child resists going and it is causing her some anxiety, it's time to reevaluate. Be your child's (and your own) advocate: remember that therapists want your child to succeed, but they may need some feedback from you. Share your experiences regarding unhelpful tactics, set boundaries about use of pressure, and give the therapist your wish list for outcomes to keep you both on the same page. If you can't come to an agreement, you can move on.

Define Goals

The following list gives an idea of what can be achieved within a trust-and-permission-based therapeutic relationship, and can provide a common language as you work with your therapist on goal-setting. Beware of timetables for goals: deadlines invite pressure.

- Help your child become more comfortable with sensations in his mouth. (This goal is especially important for therapies focused on improving sensorimotor tolerance and responses.)

- Identify and work on oral motor delays.

- Help your child determine appropriate motor response based on sensory input of food.

- Let your child determine the pace and help you read cues for readiness to transition to new foods.

- Allow your child opportunities to try new foods in a safe, nonthreatening way with a new person.

- Seek multidisciplinary referrals to address any contributing problems.

- Get physical or occupational therapy help with gross motor skills (such as sitting without fatigue) or fine motor skills (such as picking up foods with fingers).

- Get help from a pediatric dietitian to support nutrition and provide guidance for supplement use. Be wary if she persists only with pushing calories, adding on fats, and so on.

Whomever you work with, the primary goal must be to keep feeding relaxed and pleasant and avoid increasing anxiety or resistance. Observe the therapist interacting with your child to see if she refrains from pressuring and can "interpret the child's stress signals to keep the oral sensorimotor practice and feeding situations pleasurable and nonstressful" (American Speech-Language-Hearing Association 2001).

Red Flags

A decade into Jenny's STEPS program at the Callier Center, she interviewed parents to formally record perceptions of prior therapies. Most complained of not understanding their child's difficulties, being left in the lobby while their child was removed for therapy, and feeling pushed to do things that felt wrong. There were few positive comments, and parents felt frustrated that the therapy they had spent time and money on didn't work or made things worse.

The last thing you want is to end up worse off. Remember that parent who talked about feeling like he was on an alien planet during therapy? Therapy shouldn't feel like that. The burden is on the therapist to provide you with a clear picture of what therapy entails, and if the therapist doesn't want to answer questions, that's a red flag. There should be a feeling of alliance, not antagonism. Bad therapy is worse than no therapy. Many of our clients express sadness that their child "failed" therapy. We suggest that therapy often fails the child.

Pressure Creeping In

When you are trying to avoid pressure at home, you don't want pressure during therapy working against you. A feeding therapist can provide your child with opportunities to try things (oral motor work, interacting with food, tasting food) without coercion. If what you are doing—even on the direction of a PhD or a feeding team at a children's hospital—increases anxiety, pressure, gagging, or vomiting, it's not helping. Taking your child to pressuring therapy undermines your child's trust in you.

"It's All Your Fault"

With some therapies, particularly behavioral therapies, a strict protocol is set up in the clinic for you to follow at home. But the clinic isn't the real world. There are no siblings or soccer games there; nor are there extra people at home preparing foods and cleaning up. So blaming the parents for lack of progress because they aren't holding the spoon correctly, using the reinforcement schedule, or adequately ignoring negative behaviors is simplistic. Reinforcements stop working; kids get bored with videos and toys. Parents tire of dragging a thrashing child to the highchair and forcing those first bites "until he gives up." Teaching your child to eat is not about breaking his spirit or getting him to give in.

Safe Foods Are Taken Away

Many children with EPE will have been happily self-feeding a handful of safe foods, but some therapists will not allow children to self-feed. They may ask parents to backtrack to feeding pureed foods from a spoon to get in more calories and assert control. To remove safe or preferred foods takes away the child's safety net and any enjoyment of eating, and increases anxiety. One mom of a three-year-old with a feeding tube was told to stop giving her daughter the finger foods she enjoyed, including chicken, celery sticks with cream cheese or peanut butter, and various crackers. The feeding team insisted

Mom only spoon-feed purees because allowing finger foods gave the child control instead of the feeder. Sounds crazy, right? It happens all the time.

Some parents who have been instructed to add butter, oils, and cream to all foods and drinks (to increase calories) find that their child's first safe foods are *plain* fruits or vegetables. One mom was thrilled when her daughter happily ate *something*—plain cucumbers. The doctor scolded the mom, telling her to "drown it in dressing" to increase calories; her sad little girl rejected the dressing-drenched cucumbers.

One of the tips and strategies we've reviewed to support progress with eating and drinking may be just what your child needs, or you might come up with something totally different that meets your child where he is. Be curious, open, and responsive to his abilities as you learn to look at old foods and habits in new ways. Whether it's your family figuring this out at home or you are working with a therapist, how you feel and how your child reacts will tell you if it's the right approach. And since your child won't suddenly eat broccoli and broiled fish (it happens, but rarely!), we will review other ways to know that you're moving in the right direction. In the next and final chapter, we will lay out how you can tell (beyond less stress and anxiety) if you are making progress. The sweet smell of success will be hard to miss!

CHAPTER 9

Steps Toward Hope and Progress

Understanding what progress looks like can help you stick with the steps and reinforce your efforts in the areas where you feel less confident. It can help to know that, initially, progress isn't even about the food. This chapter identifies the stages of progress and what to look for. One child's progress may follow that stepwise trajectory from first getting comfortable in the same room with a challenging food, to sitting calmly at the table with it, to putting it on her plate, to touching it with a fork, and sometime later to eating it. Another child will wait and wait, not trying anything new for months. Then suddenly he will serve himself, taste, and decide he likes a new food. Neither way is wrong.

Take riding a bicycle. One child struggles for weeks, picking herself up over and over, while another waits, perhaps until she is far older, and learns to ride in an afternoon. Children with autism or younger children may simply need to be free to make a shift in the way they think about what eating is and isn't (Nadon, Feldman, and Gisel 2013).

One mom summarized a year of progress: "When we stopped pushing and enjoyed meals together, he began to eat more of his safe foods and pretty quickly started to gain weight. That was great, but he also turned into this happy kid; he was even sleeping better. Recently he asked for lettuce on his sandwich. It's such a relief to see him enjoy something green!" We often can't predict or understand why children do what they do or when. Every child's path and progress is unique. But, as the saying goes, the proof is in the pudding!

Generally, children progress more quickly when they are younger, have less severe medical, oral motor, or sensory challenges, or have experienced less pressure and anxiety around food. Whatever the child's age, however, progress around eating is not a steady march. Interest in or actual trying of new foods ebbs and flows; there may be a few days where that window feels open, only to slam shut again when a friend or teacher makes a comment, when a food turns out to be too challenging, or for no apparent reason. When you see progress, be careful not to come on too strong. We have heard from overjoyed parents that a child tried pasta salad at a picnic, and on the way home they bought several kinds of pasta salad only to have the child refuse it again for months. Be prepared to wait again or to feel disappointed after a breakthrough. Rushing the process can be counterproductive.

Long-Term vs. Short-Term Goals

The long-term goal is to raise a child who feels good about food and can eat a variety of foods based on internal cues of hunger and fullness. (Remember that "variety" doesn't have to include sushi and kale, but should consist of enough foods to meet the child's nutritional needs.) A short-term goal might be to have enjoyable family meals, or for your child to come to the table happily. Defining your goals in terms of these categories can help protect you from slipping back into pressuring. If, for example, you can table your concern about improving nutrition and recognize it as a *long-term* goal, that can help you focus on more immediate goals and progress.

Here are some sample short-term goals:

- Sits comfortably at the table

- Shows decreased anxiety around foods

- Shows increased familiarity with a variety of foods

- Shows decreased anxiety around eating out

And here are some sample long-term goals:

- Eats more balanced meals

- Can tune in to hunger cues

- Gets back on his growth curve

- Improves his nutrition

- Attends sleepaway camp

Progress in Oral Motor or Sensory Skills

As your child progresses, he will learn how to move his tongue more precisely within his mouth, respond to the sensory properties of foods with appropriate motor movements, and chew more completely. He might drool or bite his tongue less often, spit food out less, or chew with his molars more. Pocketing (keeping food in the cheeks) and gagging will decrease. He'll eventually remain calm when food gets on him, will eat new textures, and will demonstrate control with utensils. Your therapist can show how your child's oral coordination and strength is changing in more subtle ways.

Mostly, you will know your child is progressing because he will gain confidence that he *can* eat new foods. His comfort and confidence will be your ultimate gauge of progress.

Stages of Progress

While the timing and details of progress differ from child to child, an overarching pattern emerges when the steps are in place. Look hard for signs of improvement. Refer to your journal, written exercises, or Food for Thought notes. Looking back on where you started—or even back a few weeks—reminds you of how far you have come. Managing your expectations once you have taken the leap is crucial so that you don't give up prematurely or rebound to a pressuring feeding practice.

We find that progress happens in stages. The distinction between the stages is somewhat artificial; you might see signs from stage 2 earlier, or stage 1 signs later, for example. We find that often parents are still so focused on bites and calories that it's hard to look up from the numbers to see the changes happening right before their eyes. While some progress will be obvious (it no longer takes two of you to wedge him into his booster seat), some will be more subtle (he doesn't ask for crackers first thing in the morning).

Stage 1: Less Stress

Usually the first positive thing parents notice is that the child's stress decreases. Older children will often tell you flat out, "I like the way we do things now," or "Can you teach Grandma our new rules? She still makes me eat all my meat before I can have dessert and I don't want to go there anymore." Other times your child won't come out and tell you, but you'll know that she is happier. You may reflect: "She's mostly eating bread and yogurt right now, which is tough, but she's much more relaxed at mealtimes."

You may still be convinced that rewarding your child with TV is the only way, or feel certain that your child will eat less and lose weight—and she might for a time, as you learned in chapter 4. Your child might eat less for anywhere from days to months, but this behavior typically resolves more quickly when you have the steps in place. As you see your child's anxiety decrease, you may begin to feel a sense of relief, experiencing decreased stress yourself and not dreading meals quite as much. You will likely still be hyperaware of how many bites are taken and of what foods. Your anxiety may even spike if your child eats less in terms of amount or variety, but some fluctuation is normal. The first few days to weeks will be the hardest, as you wait for those first glimmers of hunger or decreased anxiety in your child.

Here are a few signs to look for, journal about, and share with your support system:

- Able to sit longer

- Not asking for the iPad as much

- Not asking for sippy cups or snacks as much

- Wakes up happier

- Sleeping better

- Decreased anxiety overall

- Less whining in the transition to meals

- Doesn't need to be dragged to the table kicking and screaming

- Less agitated or fidgety

- Better behaved

- More willing to help prepare food

- Asks about food

- Serves food onto plate, though doesn't touch it

Stage 1 lays the foundation for all progress that follows. The decrease in anxiety and increase in comfort and ease around food allows your child's internal motivation to emerge and hunger and appetite cues to be heard. Stage 1 is most defined by this decrease in anxiety, hopefully for both you and your child. While you will surely feel that you are making "mistakes," stage 1—for you—is about figuring out the steps, guided by your child's reactions. One mom reflected: "What a relief it is not to be the food cop anymore. I feel like a mom for the first time in a long time—that I can actually enjoy sitting and eating with my child is a revelation—even if it is buttered noodles and toast for now."

Stage 1 is also when your child will test the new rules most vigorously. He may eat less, even dropping a safe food or eating nothing for a meal to see if you will slip back to bribing or begging. *Hang in there! This is normal. He is testing you.* He needs to know if you really mean it when you say that he doesn't have to lick or taste something, or that he can have his dessert first.

Knowing this is coming, you will be better able to ride out the storm. Learning as much as you can, having your support in place, and addressing your anxieties before you dive in gives you the best chance for success. If you recognize that you jumped without your parachute and slipped back into pressuring, don't panic. You can get back to the steps. Though starting and stopping may slow the process of your child trusting you and the new approach, it won't do irreparable damage.

Stage 2: Increasing Comfort

In stage 2 *you* may be able to eat more calmly, feel more confident, have more ideas about how to present foods, and make better decisions over time and in the moment. You might see more progress from your child, first in terms of appetite and amounts eaten, and then in terms of variety. You'll note a few larger meals or snacks, and decreased panic at the sight of trigger foods. You may also notice your child is:

- Asking for seconds or more for the first time

- Saying "I'm hungry" for the first time, or more often

- More open to trying new desserts, like a new flavor of ice cream

- More open to eating out or less fearful of coming to the table

- Engaging in conversation more at the table

- Engaging in cooking more, expressing interest in foods

- Using utensils more appropriately

- Engaged with family

- Talking happily

- Sitting nicely

- Serving herself or others

- Commenting on her food or others'

- Playing with food: biting toast into shapes, playing with noodles, making hills out of mashed potatoes

We've heard: "The other day, he was excited to see canned peaches he recognized from Grandma's. He didn't eat them, but he was chatting about them with a lightness we hadn't seen before." And: "I can't believe it! He just asked for and dipped bread into squash soup! I was giving up hope that he would ever branch out; I was just thrilled that he was happier and more confident. It took months, but I have even more hope now!"

Stage 3: Greater Confidence

Stage 3 is generally more of what you see in stage 2, just more often and reliably. Your child will likely be steadily adding new foods to his repertoire, and perhaps will begin expressing interest in cooking or preparing food with you. You'll see:

- Bigger meals, more often

- An attitude that's reliably neutral or nonchalant around new foods

- The ability to say, "No, thank you"

Your child may still "regress" in terms of variety at times. Hang in there. You are planting seeds, and it takes a while for them to grow.

You will continue to gain confidence as you see your child continue to tune in to hunger and fullness cues and come to the table happier. Soon, you'll wonder how you did things any other way. Your child may be in stage 3 for months or years. In fact, he may continue to expand his tastes well into adulthood.

We've heard parents in this stage remark: "I was very picky until my teens, and in my thirties I am still finding new foods I like. He's only six, and I don't have to feel bad that he isn't eating tofu right now." And "Eating crunchy foods had been his last hurdle and it seems we are making it. He is eating crackers along with chicken nuggets and cupcakes at birthday parties, samples at stores, banana chunks that aren't mashed...it feels like a miracle. If he could go from being hand-fed baby food to eating functionally in eighteen months of hard work, any child can."

When Progress Stalls or Reverses

Sometimes progress comes in bursts, as with language or gross motor skills. Sometimes your child may suddenly regress back to safe foods, or eat less for a time. Rather than thinking of this as a negative or being stuck, you can think of it as a rest or pause, or a gathering of momentum or interest. In a 2007 article, Marsha Dunn Klein talks about this phenomenon as a "plateau" that can last for several months. Some therapists say this means the child needs another round of therapy, and while that is an option, waiting and supporting often works.

> **Food for Thought:** What else is happening in your child's life? Is he starting a new school or awaiting a new sibling? Is he having trouble with a friend? Is he being teased about his eating? Is a teacher or family member pushing him? Is he sleeping well? Are early puberty hormones making her more emotional?

Falling Back into Old Patterns

Sometimes progress stalls because old patterns are hard to break and parents may still be participating in counterproductive feeding practices. Be prepared to feel lured back into pressure tactics, or to be told by a new doctor or therapist to use pressure. Particularly for school-aged children who want to be like their friends, this can be challenging. They will tell you they want to push themselves, and will seem enthusiastic about schemes for trying new foods. Several children we've helped even pestered parents for sticker charts or food journals recommended by the new pediatrician or therapist. With almost all of these attempts, parents and children were disappointed when, faced with the new food and blank journal page, the child dissolved in tears, gagging or getting down only one bite over forty-five minutes. If this happens, you might say: **"We can try the food-tasting journal. It's up to you. If you want to rate foods, it could be fun, but know that we trust you'll figure this out when the time is right, and if you feel rushed or unhappy, we'll stop."**

Still Pressuring

As the proverb says, "Every slip is not a fall." It is hard to let go of tactics that worked to get in a few bites of veggies or sips of supplement. It can be especially difficult when there appears to be a valid reason for pressuring, like chronic constipation or poor weight gain. Sometimes clients say, "The steps aren't working!" Often progress stalls when parents are doing some steps, but not others: still bribing with dessert, still lecturing, still spoon-feeding every bite, still pressuring, begging, or taking the child to pressuring therapy. Even with all the steps in place, the last bit of pressure may be what is said, and it can be so subtle that parents are often surprised when we point out how certain comments are perceived as pressure.

One mom said: "I realized I was still talking about food and trying to get Cooper to cook and touch foods with me. I tried to make it fun, but it wasn't working. When I paid attention to his body

209

language and what he was telling me, I stopped making food a big deal at all."

Still Bribing with Dessert

Bribing with dessert is the tactic that parents most commonly cling to. Serving dessert after the meal is so ingrained that dangling the dessert in front of the child to shape their eating feels natural. Add in other adults who think they are helping by holding back dessert until your child eats something "healthy," and it is easy to see why parents are reluctant to change this practice. You are human, and no matter how determined you are, you can still be swayed by others who care for or are around your child. Consider how continuing to bribe with dessert sabotages your plans, and review the section on sweets and treats in chapter 7 to refresh your memory (and resolve!) when you are tempted.

Finding Your Own Pace

Maybe you haven't gotten all the steps down yet. We get it. Sometimes, it's all you can do to get out the door in the morning. One approach to lingering challenges, like feeling stuck only serving a favorite food in front of the TV for every snack, is to rip off the Band-Aid and commit to following all the steps: get in the groove of serving meals and snacks at the table without distractions and stick with a routine for several months. Once you see progress and are comfortable with the steps, then you can add a snack or two a week in front of the TV, or be more flexible with the routine on weekends.

Making smaller changes and progressing slowly is also a fine way to do things; snack is still in front of the TV after school when your child needs to unwind, but begin to offer new foods with favorites. Or continue to pack all safe foods in a lunchbox for now and work on removing the iPad at dinner. This is a reminder to find the approach that works for your family.

Deadlines Undermine Progress

Sometimes a parent tells us, "We've agreed to try this until Halloween." But you might be selling yourself (and your child) short if you have a deadline for STEPS+. All too often, the deadline approaches while the parent is still learning how not to pressure, or hasn't quite gotten hold of the routine and is still catering. It can take months to get this all down. If your son has to eat "twenty foods by Halloween," you might stop using the steps just as your child is beginning to form new neural pathways and get out of that rut of fear around food. It would be such a shame to not give it enough time, and to reinstate the same feeding practices that helped make those ruts and patterns in the first place. Deadlines also invite an agenda to the table, rather than a focus on providing a supportive experience, and the agenda invites pressure.

When You Feel Stuck

If you are still feeling conflicted, confused, or unable to make changes, you may need to think about how your own challenges may hinder this process. If you are struggling, it will be hard to help your child.

Feeling Stuck with Your Own Eating

If you have conflicted feelings about eating or your weight, as many adults do, and this is holding back progress for your family, find help. Help is available for all such conditions, from active eating disorders to more typical disordered eating where thinking about eating and your weight takes the pleasure out of your life. We've also seen parents motivated by a child's success, as this mother was: "I am seeing my daughter eat in an amazing way; feeling hungry, stopping even in the middle of a favorite food when she's had enough, and she's getting back on the growth curve! If she can do it, maybe I can learn to trust my body too?"

Feeling Stuck with Your Anxiety

If you feel as if your child is making progress, but your own anxiety is overwhelming, you may be stuck in some wagon rut neural pathways: that automatic response of dread, even when you know better. Parenting is one of the most potent triggers for our own past—joyful, sorrowful, or traumatic. If you feel stuck with anxiety or depression, get help. If you suspect you might have obsessive-compulsive disorder (OCD), generalized anxiety, or lingering post-partum depression, find treatment and support.

One mom suffered from OCD, and since the birth of her child, the focus of her obsessive thoughts had been on what her son ate. By working through the steps, she was able to tell when her thinking was part of her OCD. She started therapy and medication while journaling and writing concrete reminders for herself, such as "Don't praise," "Michael can do it," and "What's my job?" and found that as her thoughts became less obsessive, the overall anxiety and conflict around food improved. Slowly, her son began to feel more comfortable and branch out.

Taking care of yourself and your adult relationships helps you take care of your child. You might consider individual, couples, or family counseling, or find a local or online support group. One mom confided: "I really needed someone to hash all this out with, but my husband couldn't listen anymore. I get it, I'm sick of it too, but I'm in the trenches. My online support group with other parents who get it gave me an outlet."

Even if your child remains selective, you can still raise a happy and healthy person. That deep knowledge can help you have the patience to support your child as he becomes the best eater he can be, at his own pace. As one mom said: "He's eating enough to meet his basic needs. Selective and happy is way better than selective and miserable. Whether or not he expands his choices is no longer what I let define him. We'll be okay either way."

Our parting words to you are these: It can and does get better. While having the privilege to walk with families on this journey, we are continuously impressed by the dedication and effort parents put into helping their children. We know you might be scared, frustrated, tired; we imagine many of you reading this book at night, kids finally in bed. But in bringing together the full range of advice, strategies, and tips we have shared with clients, our goal is for you to feel understood, supported, relieved, and empowered. We hope that you will feel better equipped, whatever your challenges may be. We hope you no longer feel so alone, have a growing understanding of your journey, and, most importantly, feel surer of your footing on the path ahead.

Be kind with yourself and with your children as you make these changes moving forward. We hope for you what we have seen for so many of our clients: not only a way beyond extreme picky eating, but a way to reconnect with your child and with the joy of parenting.

References

More resources and recommended reading are available online at http://www.newharbinger.com/31106.

Andaya, A. A., E. M. Arredondo, J. E. Alcaraz, S. P. Lindsay, and J. P. Elder. 2011. "The Association Between Family Meals, TV Viewing During Meals, and Fruit, Vegetables, Soda, and Chips Intake Among Latino Children." *Journal of Nutrition Education and Behavior* 43(5): 308–15.

American Speech-Language-Hearing Association. 2001. *Roles of Speech-Language Pathologists in Swallowing and Feeding Disorders: Technical Report.* Rockville, MD: ASHLA.

Bartoshuk, L. M., V. B. Duffy, and I. J. Miller. 1994. "PTC/PROP Tasting: Anatomy, Psychophysics, and Sex Effects." *Physiology and Behavior* 56(6): 1165–71.

Batsell, W. R. Jr., A. S. Brown, M. E. Ansfield, and G. Y. Paschall. 2002. "'You Will Eat All of That!' A Retrospective Analysis of Forced Consumption Episodes." *Appetite* 38(3): 211–19.

Beers, D. 2009. "Michael Pollan, Garden Fresh." *The Tyee,* June 12.

Benton, D. 2010. "The Plausibility of Sugar Addiction and Its Role in Obesity and Eating Disorders." *Journal of Clinical Nutrition* 29: 288–303.

Black, M. M., and F. E. Aboud. 2011. "Responsive Feeding Is Embedded in a Theoretical Framework of Responsive Parenting." *Journal of Nutrition* 141(3): 490–94.

Chatoor, I. 2009. *Diagnosis and Treatment of Feeding Disorders in Infants, Toddlers, and Young Children.* Washington, DC: Zero to Three.

Coldwell, S. E., T. K. Oswald, and D. R. Reed. 2009. "A Marker of Growth Differs Between Adolescents with High Versus Low Sugar Preference." *Physiology and Behavior* 96(4–5): 574–80.

Crum, A. J., W. R. Corbin, K. D. Brownell, and P. Salovey. 2011. "Mind over Milkshakes: Mindsets, Not Just Nutrients, Determine Ghrelin Response." *Health Psychology* 30(4): 424–29.

Didehbani, N., K. Kelly, L. Austin, and A. Wiechmann. 2011. "Role of Parental Stress on Pediatric Feeding Disorders." *Children's Health Care* 40: 85–100.

Faber, A., and E. Mazlish. 2012. *How to Talk So Kids Will Listen and Listen So Kids Will Talk.* New York: Scribner.

Farrow, C., and H. Coulthard. 2012. "Relationships Between Sensory Sensitivity, Anxiety and Selective Eating in Children." *Appetite* 58(3): 842–46.

Fay, J., and C. Fay. 2000. *Love and Logic Magic for Early Childhood: Practical Parenting from Birth to Six Years.* Golden, CO: Love and Logic Press.

Fisher, J. O., and L. L. Birch. 2000. "Parents' Restrictive Feeding Practices Are Associated with Young Girls' Negative Self-Evaluation of Eating." *Journal of the American Dietetic Association* 100(11): 1341–46.

Fraker, C., M. Fishbein, S. Cox, and L. Walbert. 2009. *Food Chaining: The Proven 6-Step Plan to Stop Picky Eating, Solve Feeding*

Problems, and Expand Your Child's Diet. Philadelphia: Da Capo Press.

Fulkerson, J. A., M. Story, D. Neumark-Sztainer, and S. Rydell. 2008. "Family Meals: Perception of Benefits and Challenges Among Parents of 8- to 10-Year-Old Children." *Journal of the American Dietetic Association* 108(4): 706–9.

Galloway, A. T., L. Fiorito, L. Francis, and L. Birch. 2006. "'Finish Your Soup': Counterproductive Effects of Pressuring Children to Eat on Intake and Affect." *Appetite* 46(3): 318–23.

Greene, R. 2010. *The Explosive Child*. New York: HarperCollins.

Harris, G., J. Blissett, and R. Johnson. 2000. "Food Refusal Associated with Illness." *Child Psychology and Psychiatry Review* 5(4): 148–56.

Klein, Marsha Dunn. 2007. "Tube Feeding Transition Plateaus." *Exceptional Parent Magazine* 37(2): 22–5.

Kotler, L. A., P. Cohen, M. Davies, D. S. Pine, and B. T. Walsh. 2011. "Longitudinal Relationships Between Childhood, Adolescent, and Adult Eating Disorders." *Journal of the American Academy of Child and Adolescent Psychiatry* 40(12): 1434–40.

Levine, M. 2012. "Raising Successful Children." *New York Times,* August 5: SR8.

Lytle, L., A. I. Eldridge, K. Kotz, J. Piper, S. Williams, and B. Kalina. 1997. "Children's Interpretation of Nutrition Messages." *Journal of Nutrition Education* 29(3): 128–36.

Maimaran, M., and A. Fishbach. 2014. "If It's Useful and You Know It, Do You Eat? Preschoolers Refrain from Instrumental Food." *Journal of Consumer Research* 41(3): 642–55.

Martin, C. I., T. M. Dovey, H. Coulthard, and A. M. Southall. 2013. "Maternal Stress and Problem-Solving Skills in a Sample of

Children with Nonorganic Feeding Disorders." *Infant Mental Health Journal* 34(3): 202–10.

Millward, C., M. Ferriter, S. J. Calver, and G. G. Connell-Jones. 2008. "Gluten- and Casein-Free Diets for Autistic Spectrum Disorder." *Cochrane Database of Systematic Reviews.* DOI: 10.1002/14651858.CD003498.pub3.

Morris, S. E. 2002. "Hemi-Sync for Learning and Stress Reduction: User's Guide." http://www.new-vis.com/fym/pdf/papers/learning .1.pdf.

Morris, S. E., and M. D. Klein. 2000. *Pre-Feeding Skills, Second Edition: A Comprehensive Resource for Mealtime Development.* Austin, TX: PRO-ED.

Murkett, T., and G. Rapley. 2010. *Baby-Led Weaning: The Essential Guide to Introducing Solid Foods and Helping Your Baby to Grow Up a Happy and Confident Eater.* New York: The Experiment.

Nadon, G., D. Feldman, and E. Gisel. 2013. "Feeding Issues Associated with the Autism Spectrum Disorders." In *Recent Advances in Autism Spectrum Disorders*, Vol. 1, edited by M. Fitzgerald. DOI:10.5772/53644.

Newman, J., and A. Taylor. 1992. "Effect of a Means-End Contingency on Young Children's Food Preferences." *Journal of Experimental Child Psychology* 53(2): 200–16.

Neumark-Sztainer, D. 2009. "Preventing Obesity and Eating Disorders in Adolescents: What Can Health Care Providers Do?" *Journal of Adolescent Health* 44(3): 206–13.

O'Dea, J. A., and R. Wilson. 2006. "Socio-Cognitive and Nutritional Factors Associated with Body Mass Index in Children and Adolescents: Possibilities for Childhood Obesity Prevention." *Health Education Research* 21(6): 796–805.

Owen, J. P., E. J. Marco, S. Desai, E. Fourie, J. Harris, S. S. Hill, A. B. Arnett, and P. Mukherjee. 2013. Abnormal White Matter Microstructure in Children with Sensory Processing Disorders. *Neuroimage: Clinical* .23(2): 844–53.

Perry, B., R. Pollard, T. Blakley, W. Baker, and D. Vigilante. 1995. "Childhood Trauma, the Neurobiology of Adaptation, and 'Use-Dependent' Development of the Brain: How 'States' Become 'Traits.'" *Infant Mental Health Journal* 16(4): 271–91.

Pinhas, L., G. McVey, K. S. Walker, M. Norris, D. Katzman, and S. Collier. 2013. "Trading Health for a Healthy Weight: The Uncharted Side of Healthy Weight Initiatives." *Eating Disorders* 21(2): 109–16.

Rowell, K. J. 2012. *Love Me, Feed Me: The Adoptive Parent's Guide to Ending the Worry About Weight, Picky Eating, Power Struggles and More.* St. Paul, MN: Family Feeding Dynamics.

Sanger, G. J., P. M. Hellstrom, and E. Naslund. 2010. "The Hungry Stomach: Physiology, Disease, and Drug Development Opportunities." *Frontiers in Pharmacology* 1: 145.

Satter, E. M. 1986. "The Feeding Relationship." *Journal of the American Dietetic Association* 86(3): 352–56.

———. 2000. *Child of Mine: Feeding with Love and Good Sense.* Boulder, CO: Bull Publishing.

———. 2014. "Avoid Pressure." http://ellynsatterinstitute.org/htf /avoidpressure.php.

Spagnola, M., and B. H. Fiese. 2007. "Family Routines and Rituals: A Context for Development in the Lives of Young Children." *Infants and Young Children* 20(4): 284–99.

Van Dyke, N., and E. J. Drinkwater. 2013. "Review Article: Relationships Between Intuitive Eating and Health Indicators: Literature Review." *Public Health Nutrition* 21: 1–10.

Van Zetten, Skye. 2013. "Feeding a Need." *Mealtime Hostage* [blog]. http://www.mealtimehostage.com/2013/07/18/feeding-a-need/

Vasylyeva, T. L., A. Barche, S. P. Chennasamudram, C. Sheehan, R. Singh, and M. E. Okogbo. 2013. "Obesity in Prematurely Born Children and Adolescents: Follow Up in Pediatric Clinic." *Nutrition Journal* 12(1): 150.

Williams, K. E., K Riegel, and M. L. Kerwin. 2009. "Feeding Disorder of Infancy or Early Childhood: How Often Is It Seen in Feeding Programs?" *Children's Health Care* 38(2): 123–36.

Woolley, H., L. Hertzmann, and A. Stein. 2007. "Video-Feedback Intervention with Mothers with Postnatal Eating Disorders and Their Infants." In *Promoting Positive Parenting: An Attachment-Based Intervention*, edited by F. Juffer, M. J. Bakermans-Kranenburg, and M. H. van IJzendoorn. New York: Routledge.

Katja Rowell, MD, is a family doctor and childhood feeding specialist on a mission to support parents who worry about feeding and their child's weight or growth. Known as "the Feeding Doctor," she is a national expert on children, feeding, and the intersection of health and wellness. Rowell believes that helping children grow up to feel good about food and their bodies is the best preventive medicine there is. Described as "academic, but warm and down to earth," she presents workshops to parents and professionals across the country. Rowell consults with a range of clients and writes on the importance of a healthy feeding relationship for online and print media. She has shared tips on how to bring peace back to meals through DVDs, TV, and radio, and is author of *Love Me, Feed Me*. Rowell makes her home in the Twin Cities, where she enjoys reading, camping, cooking (most of the time) for her family, and a husband who does the dishes.

Jenny McGlothlin, MS, CCC-SLP, is a certified speech-language pathologist specializing in the evaluation and treatment of feeding disorders for children from birth through the teen years. McGlothlin developed the STEPS feeding program at the Callier Center for Communication Disorders at University of Texas at Dallas, where she works with families on a daily basis to foster feeding skills that will serve a child for a lifetime. Her passion is teaching children how to eat when they just can't figure it out on their own, and McGlothlin has been inducted into the Texas Speech-Language-Hearing Association's Hall of Fame for her work in the field. McGlothlin has spent many years teaching graduate-level courses on feeding as well as early child development. She frequently provides feeding workshops for parents and continuing education seminars and webinars for therapists. As a mother of three young children, McGlothlin makes family meals a priority, and enjoys reading and spending time with her friends.

Foreword writer **Suzanne Evans Morris, PhD**, is an internationally recognized speaker and therapist for infants and children with feeding and mealtime challenges. With more than fifty years' experience as a speech-language pathologist specializing in feeding development and disorders in children, she pioneered the development of feeding and mealtime programs in the United States. Morris is coauthor of three books: *Pre-Feeding Skills*, the *Mealtime Participation Guide*, and the *Homemade Blended Formula Handbook*.

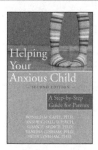
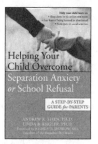
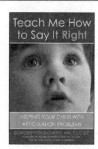
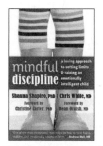
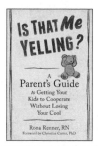
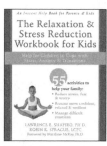

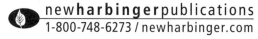

Register your **new harbinger** titles for additional benefits!

When you register your **new harbinger** title—purchased in any format, from any source—you get access to benefits like the following:

- Downloadable accessories like printable worksheets and extra content

- Instructional videos and audio files

- Information about updates, corrections, and new editions

Not every title has accessories, but we're adding new material all the time.

Access free accessories in 3 easy steps:

1. Sign in at NewHarbinger.com (or **register** to create an account).

2. Click on **register a book**. Search for your title and click the **register** button when it appears.

3. Click on the **book cover or title** to go to its details page. Click on **accessories** to view and access files.

That's all there is to it!

If you need help, visit:

NewHarbinger.com/accessories

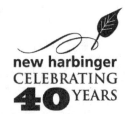

new harbinger
CELEBRATING
40 YEARS